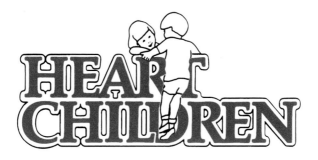

A Practical Handbook for parents of children with congenital heart problems

This book is dedicated
to Heart Children and their parents
everywhere ...but especially
in joyful remembrance of
Esther Clark aged 21,
of Camberley, Surrey,
whose courage and sheer love of life
was an inspiration to us all.

FOREWORD
Making sense of it all

The purpose of this book is to help you deal with some of the feelings and problems that come your way as you live with a child who has a heart problem. It is also to provide medical information in a way that can be understood by parents and others with a non-clinical background. The authors would like to stress that this book in *no way* replaces information received from your hospital, cardiologist or other clinical adviser.

You may be familiar with the feelings mentioned already – in which case, you have trodden the same path as the parents who contributed to this book. You may have experienced with us the struggle to try and make sense of it all.

You will have learned that each child's condition is different from any other and that some conditions are minor while others cannot be corrected. Some children die while others with similar conditions live.

You will become aware, if you are not already, that there are no stock answers to guide you through the difficult times. We hope we can help you come to terms with your feelings and channel them positively as you move through all the emotions and experiences that your child will bring you. We hope this book will help you to be able to cope with – and actually enjoy your life with your child who has a heart problem.

CLINICAL BACKGROUND

The majority of children with heart disease in developed countries have what is called congenital heart disease, that is, their hearts have developed abnormally early on in pregnancy. One in one hundred and twenty five of all children born in Britain have this form of heart problem. Some may be very minor and never require treatment, others may be mild and need occasional follow-up, others may be serious, requiring major operations, and a few are so serious that no treatment is currently available. The possibility of treatment has improved enormously over the last 30 years, and the majority of children, even those with very serious problems, may now be treated very successfully.

Sometimes a previously normal heart can be affected by inflammation or infection, for example, rheumatic fever, Kawasaki disease, myocarditis, endocarditis and these are conditions to which we refer in this volume.

6000567231

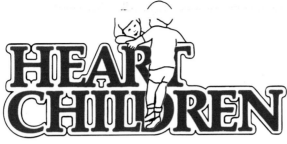

A Practical Handbook for parents of children with congenital heart problems

HeartLine Association
Community Link, Surrey Heath House, Knoll Road,
Camberley, Surrey GU15 3HD
'Heart Children: A Practical Handbook for Parents'
3rd.e. (pbk)
ISBN 0-9515270-2-9
© 1989, 1992 and 2002 HeartLine Association

1st printed September 1989 (6M)
2nd Edition January 1992 (20M)
3rd Edition March 2002 (20M)

Written by Philip Rees, Adelaide Tunstill, Tricia Pope and David Kinnear

Published for HeartLine by DK Creative Services, Camberley, Surrey, GU15 1DB, UK

Printed by Kent Edwards Litho, Bordon, Hants.

HeartLine Association is a registered charity, number 295803

ACKNOWLEDGEMENTS

HeartLine Association would like to thank **Linda Davies** and **Michelle Mann** whose own 'heart' children, **Robert** and **Jessica**, were the inspiration to write the booklet of the same title which was published in their memory in New Zealand some years ago.

HeartLine Association gladly acknowledges that many ideas from their original booklet have been incorporated into this volume for the benefit of 'heart' children and their parents everywhere.

The authors would also specially like to thank the following for their vital contribution to the preparation of this book:

- Gillian Oliver for the illustrations.
- Joyce Chu for the delightful cartoons.
- Emma Kinnear who word processed the manuscript.
- Photographs used by courtesy of the Medical Illustration Department at Great Ormond Street Hospital for Children, London.
- Russel West LRPS who prepared the scans.
- David Holt of David Holt Studios, Godalming, for design and typography, Lynda Horton, Pat and Ian Coupland of Imagination, Camberley, all of whom gave enormous help with the production of the third edition of this book.
- Frimley and Camberley Schools of Ballet who donated the proceeds of many performances to HeartLine Association.
- Eileen Clark, for her tireless and enthusiastic fundraising without which the conception of this book would not have been possible.
- The Compassionate Friends.
- The Clarissa Norman Fund.
- Patrick Ward of Rapid Print, Houghton Regis, Beds (the original printer of this book) who gave great support and technical help at the concept of the project.
- Messrs Vodafone whose generous support helped us publish the 3rd edition of this book.
- Our friends and sister organisation The Association for Children with Heart Disorders.

... and also to Tony Pope, Gill Rees and Patsy Kinnear, who have provided unfailing support and encouragement throughout the project.

ABOUT THE WRITERS

Heart Children **has been written by four people who have practical experience on the subject from first hand knowledge:**

Philip Rees   is Consultant Pediatric Cardiologist at The Great Ormond Street Hospital for Children, London and is a familiar figure to very many parents.

Adelaide Tunstill   was for many years the senior nurse in charge at the Cardiac Unit at The Great Ormond Street Hospital for Children, London, and now works with young adult patients with congenital heart disease at the Heart Hospital, University College London Hospitals. Adelaide is universally acknowledged for her experience and expertise on the subject by doctors, nurses and parents.

Tricia Pope   who is a parent member of HeartLine Association, had the idea of preparing the original book. Tricia's son, Simon, now aged 24, was born with a congenital heart disorder.

David Kinnear   who also published this book, was the first parent Chairman of Heart Line Association, and has two daughters, Emma aged 26 and Annabel aged 19, who were both born with severe heart problems.

ABOUT THIS BOOK

This completely revised and updated book, like the first and second editions before it, is written both for the parents of children with heart disease – and for the children and young adults themselves.

The impetus to prepare it came from seeing **Linda Davies** and **Michelle Mann's** lucid *'Heart Children'* booklet from New Zealand.

Further encouragement came from the **Danish Heart Foundation** booklet, *'Congenital Heart Defects'* – and also from the excellent handouts that **Doctors Olive Scott** and **Leon Gerlis** and the **British Heart Foundation** had prepared over the past few years.

The book is designed to improve knowledge and understanding. It is an outline and many generalisations have had to be made. What it does not do, is to replace the personal contact between your family and the teams involved in your child's care. PLEASE DON'T BE AFRAID TO ASK QUESTIONS of the team looking after your child – so that you have a good understanding of the problems and plans.

We have used the term 'Heart Child' for convenience as many of we parents do. This does not mean to belittle or diminish in any way our children as individuals who happen to have a heart abnormality. Our aim is for our children to grow up as normally as possible. In the text, we have used 'he' or 'him' rather than both 'he' and 'she', again for convenience. These terms can be replaced by 'she' and 'her'.

Please note also, that there are many grey zones in medicine in which the decisions made concerning your child, and the actions taken, may not follow the outline of this book, so do not be alarmed if what you read here, differs from your own experience.

PUBLISHER'S STATEMENT

Whilst this book has been prepared on the basis of information that the authors believe to be accurate, those who are in any doubt about the medical condition of their child must consult their registered medical practitioner. The authors and publishers accept no responsibility in whatever circumstances for the actions or omissions of others occasioned by their reading this book.

COPYRIGHT WARNING

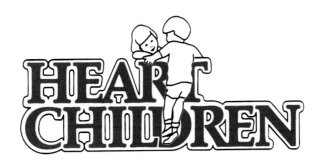

Contents

Chapter   Page

THE NORMAL HEART
Its circulation and development

The heart and lungs are positioned in the chest protected by the breast bone *(sternum)*, rib cage and spine. The heart is partly surrounded by the lungs. In small children, the thymus gland is large and lies in front of the large vessels and upper part of the heart. The heart is a pump with four chambers within it: the two (left and right) atria, and the two (left and right)ventricles. Its purpose is to pump blood that has been to the body, and given up its oxygen to the various organs, into the lungs to pick up more oxygen, and then to return this oxygenated blood into the body to supply the organs with oxygen and nutrition.

Blood returns from the body in veins. These join together to form two large veins, one from the top half of the body *(the superior vena cava)* and one from the bottom half of the body *(the inferior vena cava)* which run into the first chamber of the heart *(the right atrium).*

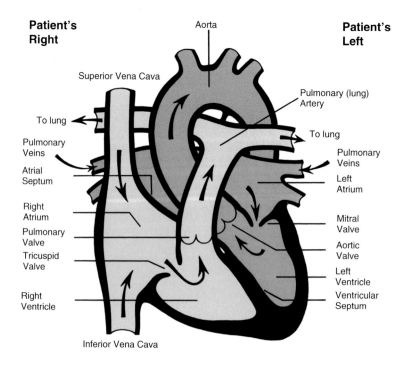

THE NORMAL HEART AND ITS CIRCULATION

This acts as a reservoir to fill the right ventricle which it does through a flap valve *(the tricuspid valve)*.

When the right ventricle contracts, this flap valve closes, the pressure in the ventricle *(pump chamber)* rises above that in the lung artery, and the pulmonary valve opens. Blood is then pumped into the lung artery and both lungs. When the ventricle starts to relax, the lung *(pulmonary)* valve closes which stops blood leaking back into the ventricle.

Within the lungs, the main arteries branch into very many small vessels which have thinner and thinner walls. They run very close to the end of the airway passages, and at this point, oxygen is taken up from the air and carbon dioxide is given off into the air passages. The blood then returns from the lungs in veins which join together, the four of these entering the receiving chamber on the left side of the heart (the left atrium). This acts as a reservoir to fill the left ventricle through another flap valve (the mitral valve). This ventricle then contracts, closing the flap valve; the pressure rises, the aortic valve opens between the left ventricle and the aorta and the blood is pumped out into the aorta. This is the large vessel that arises from the heart, and divides into the many vessels that supply the whole of the

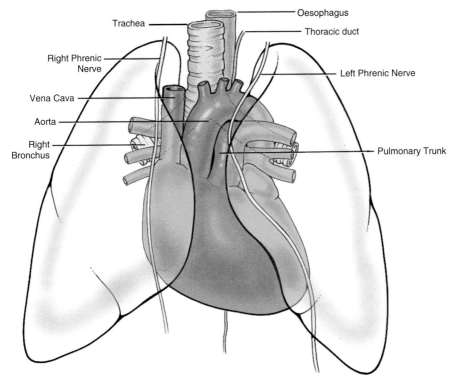

NORMAL POSITION OF HEART AND LUNGS IN THE CHEST

body. Following this, the ventricle relaxes and the aortic valve closes. During relaxation of the ventricles the mitral and tricuspid valves open and blood flows into them in preparation for the next contraction.

This process of contraction followed by relaxation occurs between 70-150 times per minute depending on the age of the patient. The heart's electrical circuit, the conduction system, controls this rate and ensures that the atria contract just before the ventricles.

The heart's own spontaneous pacemaker *(the sinus node)* is at the top right hand corner of the right atrium, see chapter 5 for more information about this. It generates an electrical impulse. This impulse (similar to what happens in a nerve) spreads through the atria causing them to contract. It then reaches the junction between the atria and the right ventricle at the *atrio-ventricular node*. There, after a short delay, the electrical signal is passed down very fast conducting fibres into both ventricles, causing them to contract.

The lungs are relatively small and have fewer and thinner walled blood vessels in comparison to those in the rest of the body. It is therefore, easier for the blood to be pumped through them.

The pressures thus generated in the right side of the heart are much less, usually a quarter, of those required by the left side of the heart to pump blood all around the body. The normal left ventricle is therefore

thick, and the normal right ventricle is thin. Both atria are thin walled, acting largely as reservoirs and only having to contract to fill the relaxed ventricles.

Heart Development

The heart muscle itself receives its blood supply from the coronary arteries which arise from the bottom of the aorta. These vessels are usually normal in children but are damaged in later life by smoking, high blood pressure, obesity and high fat diets.

The heart develops from a small group of cells in the upper part of the chest of the very small embryo. These cells rapidly form a tube and the tube folds over on itself into an 'S' shape. Bulges develop on this tube and these form the chambers of the heart and the first part of the major arteries. Between these bulges are waists. It is here that the valves develop. The heart is divided into left and right sides by walls or 'septa'. The septa grow between the two atria, the two ventricles, and also separate the two arteries.

The heart connects up with the simultaneously developing blood vessels in the body, and those within the lungs. This process is complete by ten weeks of pregnancy, following which the heart and the blood vessels just grow with the developing baby.

Circulation before birth

Before birth the *placenta* (after-birth) is the organ that supplies the baby with oxygen and nutrition and removes carbon dioxide. The lungs are not expanded and require only a small blood supply to allow them to grow. Nature has devised several short circuits to allow the most efficient use of blood flow whilst in the womb.

The oxygenated blood from the placenta returns to the inferior vena cava in the umbilical vein, and then is directed by a flap valve *(Eustachian valve)* towards the

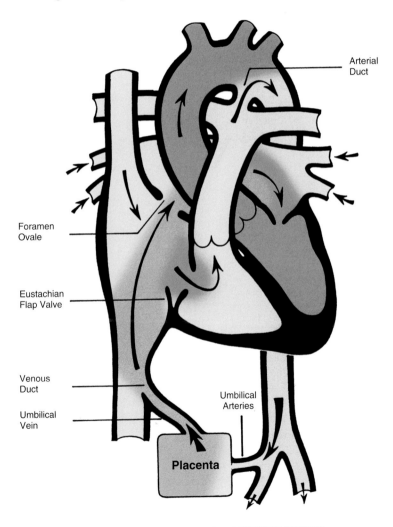

CIRCULATION BEFORE BIRTH

small hole (*foramen ovale*) between the two receiving chambers. This oxygenated blood is then pumped by the left ventricle into the aorta and up to the developing brain.

The de-oxygenated blood from the top half of the body is directed to the right ventricle which pumps it into the lung artery. The majority of the blood then goes into a tube (the duct) down the aorta into the abdomen from where the arteries arise that feed the placenta.

It is because of these connections and with the placenta in the circuit, that the majority of babies even with very major heart problems will often be apparently fine and grow normally within the womb.

Changes at birth and in the following few days

The placenta is removed from the baby's circulation as soon as the umbilical cord is clamped. The baby's lungs expand with crying and blood passes into them in increasing amounts.

The blood picks up the oxygen from the air, and the increased amount of blood returning to the left atrium closes the hole between the two atria.

Over the next few days, the tube between the two arteries gradually closes. These changes result in an increased amount of oxygen being available to the child as a

result of the lungs working. The blood pressure in the body increases, and gradually over the subsequent days and weeks, that in the lungs and in the right ventricle, falls.

Babies with significant heart problems may first show something abnormal when these changes in the circulation occur.

Notes ✐

2 | FINDING OUT WHAT'S WRONG
Examinations and investigations

The doctor will ask questions concerning your child's activity in comparison to other children of the same age, for example, feeding pattern in babies, sleeping pattern in the day time in toddlers, physical activity of children at play and at school and whether there are any activities that bring on intermittent complaints (symptoms).

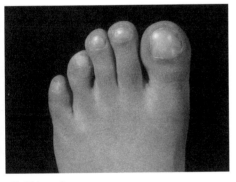

Clubbing of toes.

The general practitioner, paediatrician or cardiologist will examine your child. They will look at his size, height and weight, the colour of lips, tongue and fingers, and the shape of his nails, which may be abnormal *(clubbing)*. They will count the child's pulse and assess its quality in the arms and the legs, and often they will measure the blood pressure. They will feel the child's abdomen to look for the size of the liver, look at the chest shape and feel the heart's action. Then with their stethoscopes they will listen to the heart sounds, and also any murmurs. Heart

sounds are the noises produced as the heart valves close and murmurs are produced by the flow of blood through the heart and large vessels.

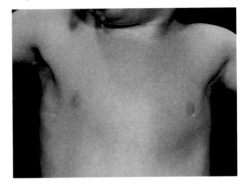

Abnormally shaped chest.

1. MURMURS

Murmurs are most frequently entirely normal coming from the normal blood flow. These are termed *'innocent'* and all is well. Other murmurs come from abnormal blood flows and may be the only sign of a problem being present.

They are often picked up during a routine examination or an incidental illness.

2. BREATHLESSNESS

Children with heart problems may often become breathless sooner than ordinary children. This occurs either because of too much or too little blood in the lungs. If too much, the lungs are heavier than normal. More effort and energy is used to expand them to move air in and out. In small children this breathlessness causes poor feeding, slow weight gain and sweating. In older children it reduces exercise tolerance. If too little blood goes to the lungs, not enough oxygen can be picked up to meet the increasing needs of the body muscles on exercise. This lack of oxygen causes an increase in the rate and depth of breathing.

3. BLUENESS

Blueness of fingers and lips can be a normal finding in normal children and relates to alterations in the blood flow and the size of the fine blood vessels of the skin and is often caused by temperature changes. Blueness of the tongue as well as fingers and toes occurs if darker blood, with less oxygen has been pumped into the body, without first passing through the lungs.

4. DIZZINESS / FAINTING

This may relate to alterations in the heart rate or to obstruction in the blood flow from the heart into the great arteries.

5. FATIGUE

Children who are blue, or whose heart muscle is working poorly, may complain of tiredness and lack of energy. This is because the muscles of the legs and arms are not receiving enough oxygenated blood.

6. SPELLS

If the muscle below the lung artery becomes thickened, it can reduce the blood flow to the lungs. The extent of the narrowing can change – when it is tight the blood flow to the

lungs falls temporarily. The amount of oxygenated blood available to the body is reduced and the child becomes bluer. This can come on suddenly without apparent reason, often after breakfast.

It is associated with a funny cry – as though in distress – restlessness, breathing difficulties followed by exhaustion and floppiness and it is termed a *'spell'*. These *spells* are usually mild to start with and settle on their own.

Over time they can become longer lasting and more serious, and it is important that your doctors are told about them.

7. SQUATTING

Blue children often squat on their haunches after walking or running. It is a normal response and increases the blood flow to the lungs by raising the blood pressure. Therefore more oxygenated blood is available and the children feel better and their colour improves. This is now much rarer than it used to be, as surgery is now undertaken earlier in life.

8. CHEST PAIN

This is very unusual in children with heart problems, and rarely comes from the heart itself, but from the muscles in the chest.

9. SUDDEN COLLAPSE

This also is **very unusual** in children's heart problems, and the vast majority of families can be reassured that this will not happen.

10. PALPITATIONS

This is the sensation of the heart beating heavily or quickly. Minor sensations are entirely normal as are extra beats. Fast heart beating, similar to the usual fast heart beat on running may come on suddenly at rest. Usually these are a nuisance and frequently children learn special tricks to slow the heart rate.

Occasionally the fast heart beat lasts for a long time causing sweatiness, paleness, breathlessness and may require specific treatment.

Investigations – the way to discover what needs to be done

Frequently, investigations are necessary to help find the exact type of heart problem that is present. Not all children will require all, or even any, of the tests described here. The decision will depend on each individual child.

ELECTROCARDIOGRAM (ECG)

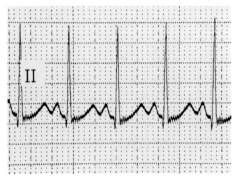

An ECG Recording.

The ECG records the faint electrical impulses which arise from the electrical circuits within the heart. It is recorded through wires and sticky patches connected to the child's arms, legs and chest. The recording is painless and takes about five minutes. It shows the heart rhythm and also may help in assessing which chambers are performing extra work.

TWENTY-FOUR HOUR ECG RECORDING

This is a recording of the electrical activity over a twenty four hour period, using a small tape recorder and wires attached to the chest. It can be undertaken as an out-patient, with the child doing normal things during the day except bathing, swimming or playing in a sand pit.

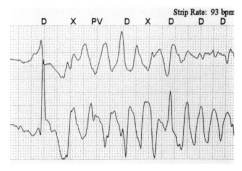

A 24 hour ECG trace showing irregular heartbeat.

This is often used when children have symptoms of fainting, dizziness or irregularities of their heart beat.

EVENT RECORDER

This is a small recording device which is attached with 2 leads onto the chest. It is able to sense the electrical activity from the heart continuously.

If symptoms occur, it can be activated and it then records the ECG for the previous 30 seconds and for the subsequent minutes. The recording can then be sent down a telephone line to a decoder and the heart rhythm analysed during these symptoms. The recorder is usually lent for between 4-6 weeks and the position of the leads can be changed every few days to allow bathing.

CHEST X-RAY

Chest X-ray shows the size and position of the heart and gives an assessment of blood flow through the lungs.

It may also show which part of the heart is enlarged.

By combining the ECG and the chest X-ray, often a very accurate diagnosis can be made.

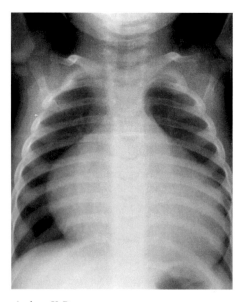

A chest X-Ray.

ECHOCARDIOGRAPHY

This uses very high pitched sound waves (sonar) to see the heart structure and assess its function.

The test is painless, although smaller children may get rather restless while it is being done and might need to be sedated. The probe, which generates the sound wave, is placed on the chest, the top of the abdomen and the neck. The sound beam is reflected back via a special computer and thence to a television screen. The pictures of the heart and its blood vessels can be seen and recorded. The direction and speed of blood flow through the circulation can be assessed by its 'Doppler' imaging system which can reproduce a colour picture of flow patterns as well as the 'whooshing' sounds of the heart and the great vessels.

(see the pictures across the page)

The improvement in both the quality of the images obtained and the assessment of the function of the heart has meant that this has now become a very accurate diagnostic investigation for children with cardiac problems. Many will no longer require catheterisation to make the diagnosis and plan appropriate care.

The tests can be done as an outpatient and take between 15 minutes and an hour, depending on the complexity of the problem.

CARDIAC CATHETERISATION AND ANGIOGRAPHY

This technique allows direct measurement of pressures within the various chambers of the heart and blood vessels. It also looks at structure and function by using a radio-opaque dye to fill part of the circulation temporarily. It is also very frequently used to treat the underlying heart problem. This involves the child coming into hospital for between 1 and 3 days. Sometimes additional tests are needed beforehand such as X-rays, ECGs and echocardiograms. These may be undertaken beforehand as an outpatient, so there is no need to be admitted until the day of the test. In some hospitals, cardiac catheterisation is done under local anaesthesia with sedation, but more frequently, it is undertaken under general anaesthesia, particularly if an interventional procedure (treatment) is being performed.

Sedatives are often given beforehand. The patient may not eat for 6 hours or drink for 4 hours before the procedure. A nurse who knows the child from the ward – and the parents too, if they wish, will bring him to the catheter room. Little children are carried and the bigger ones travel on a trolley. The family will leave when the child has settled or has been anaesthetised. The child lies on a flat table connected to

an ECG machine and an X-ray machine, which will allow the heart action to be filmed. Doctors and nurses wear special trousers, shirts, hats, gloves and put on masks to keep clean. The catheter is a fine tube, inserted usually through a needle, or occasionally through a small incision, into a vein or artery at the top of the leg. Sometimes the catheter may be inserted in the arm, or the lower part of the neck or shoulder. Then, by gently manipulating the catheter, it moves along with the blood flow through the big blood vessels and the various chambers of the heart. This enables the pressures to be measured within the various arteries. Small samples of blood may also be taken from various parts of the circulation. This shows whether there are any significant holes between the various parts of the system, and which chambers are not working properly. A radio-opaque

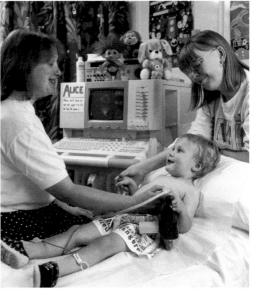

Above: A young patient having a colour Doppler scan.

Below: *the picture it makes.*

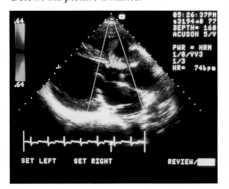

liquid (which is visible to X-rays) can also be injected down the catheter tubes to show the heart's structure on a television screen, so the clinical team can see how well it is working and whether there is any abnormality.

The cardiac catheterisation test can also be used to treat heart problems, for example, stretching narrow valves, arteries or veins, or making holes to improve the way the blood flows through the circulation or blocking abnormal

vessels and connections. This means that some operations may be avoided.

Cardiac catheterisation takes between one and three hours depending on the complexity of the case. Following this, the child will be sleepy for a few hours before returning to normal. Sometimes he is able to be discharged the same night, but more often, the following day. Although the test is a complex one, it can in the majority of children be performed very safely without problems.

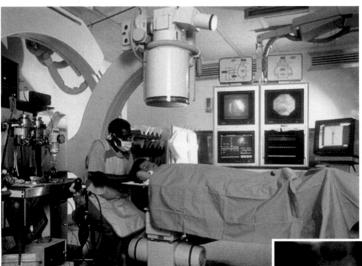

The Catheter Room. The large machine with the white drum above the patient, makes special X-ray movie pictures of the insde of the heart, so the doctors can see what is happening.

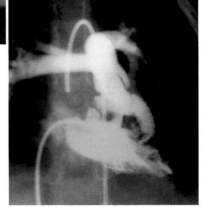

Right: *The thin white lines are the catheters.*

Other techniques

RADIO-ISOTOPE SCANNING

An injection of a very small dose of an isotope can be used either to assess the function of the heart muscle or the extra amount of blood going through lungs in children who have holes between the two sides of the circulation. This can be done at an out-patient clinic. A small injection is given, after which the child has to lie still on a special table for a short while.

ELECTROPHYSIOLOGICAL STUDIES

Children who have repeated problems from abnormalities of heart rate and rhythm, may require more detailed investigations to understand and to treat the abnormal electrical circuitry within the heart. Usually, with general anaesthesia, several fine electrical wires are steered into different parts of the circulation. The electrical activity from those local areas inside the heart are recorded directly. The different areas can be stimulated by small electrical signals passed down the wires in an attempt to bring on the abnormal heart rhythm in order to understand it better, to see how it starts and stops and in many cases, to try to remove the abnormal circuit by using radio frequency energy to modify that small area of abnormal heart tissue (called an ablation). See page 50 for more details.

The test is similar to a catheter test, but it may take up to 4-5 hours and usually involves admission to hospital for two nights. Anti-arrhythmic medicines are usually stopped five days beforehand and hopefully, do not need to be restarted after the procedure if an ablation has been successful. Frequent extra beats are common in the subsequent weeks but hopefully, no recurrence of the fast heart rate will occur.

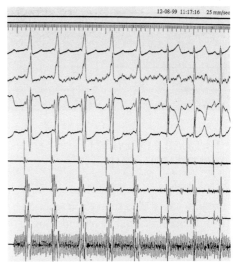

ECG recording from within the heart during ablation. Notice the changes to the ECG shapes in the top four traces. Radio frequency energy is shown by the bottom trace.

TRANSOESOPHAGEAL ECHOCARDIOGRAPHY

This is used to look at the back of the heart from the gullet (oesophagus). It is often used in adolescents and young adults when the usual echo pictures may not be so clear. It is used to assess valve function and also to look at holes in the walls between the atria and abnormal flow patterns in the lung veins. It is undertaken either under heavy sedation or under general anaesthesia and may be combined with a catheter test.

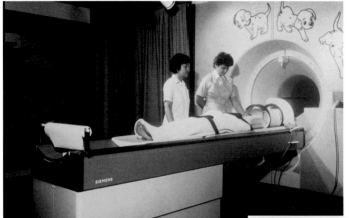

NUCLEAR MAGNETIC RESONANCE (NMR)

This involves placing the child in a large machine which uses a strong magnetic field. Images are produced by looking at the alteration of electrical forces in different parts of the body. It is possible to see the heart and other parts of the body extremely clearly and to measure blood flow very accurately. It involves lying very still in quite an enclosed space, rather like a torpedo tube, for a long time. For this reason, smaller children usually have this test done under full anaesthetic.

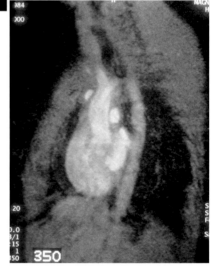

An NMR image of the side of the chest.

The images produced are particularly helpful in the adolescent and young adult with complex problems as these may be more difficult to assess with echocardiography. It is likely that developments in this field will be very dramatic over the next decade.

BARIUM SWALLOW

The child's oesophagus (food pipe) can be seen on a television picture using X-rays while drinking a sort of thick 'milk shake' containing a substance called barium. If there is any narrowing of the oesophagus or main windpipe (the trachea) caused by an abnormal blood vessel, this can usually be seen clearly with this test.

HAEMOGLOBIN

This is the chemical in the red blood cells that carries oxygen and carbon dioxide around the body. The amount present can be easily measured by a simple blood test. It is useful to check this occasionally to ensure that the level is correct, not too low, not too high for the child's condition. In blue children the level is usually higher than normal which is an advantage.

However the level should not be allowed to become too high as the blood is then very thick and flows sluggishly. When this happens operations may be advised even if the child is otherwise well. If operations are not possible some of the thick blood may be removed and replaced by a salt solution in order to dilute it.

OXYGEN SATURATION

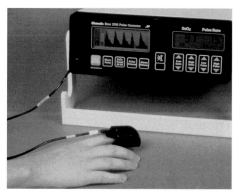

Oxygen saturation probe.

The percentage of haemoglobin that is carrying oxygen to the tissues of the body can be measured directly with a simple probe that is attached to a finger or an ear lobe. This is a painless, simple and reliable test.

EXERCISE TEST

This is used to measure the function of the heart with exercise, while recording the ECG and blood pressure. It can be done with a bicycle or a tread mill, as in the picture. It is useful to judge the reserves of the heart muscle, examine the effect of blood flow on the pump chambers, check for arrhythmias and occasionally to look for the lack of blood supply to the heart muscle (ischaemia) in producing chest pain.

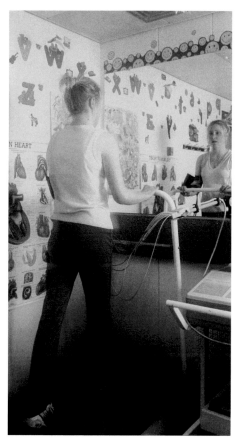

The Exercise Test is used to see how the heart is working under physical activity.

3 SPECIFIC HEART PROBLEMS
What's wrong and how they're put right

Introduction

There are many types of heart abnormalities and the more common ones are described in this chapter. Some children have more than one problem with their heart and perhaps more than one diagram will then be relevant to that child. Do not worry if your child's condition is not specifically described here – your doctors will describe the problem clearly to you. **NB.** You may find it helpful to ask them to explain by using the fold out flap and blank diagrams at the back of this book.

INNOCENT MURMURS

These normal noises are extremely common in children. Up to a quarter (25%) of healthy children have these soft *murmurs* at different times.

The *murmurs* arise from the blood flow through the large veins as they return to the chest or from the blood flow around the bends of the heart. The heart in children is compact, the normal bends are quite tight and the heart rate is faster than in adults. As a result the normal flow produces a soft noise or a *murmur*. An analogy is the noise that water makes in a stream as it curves round a bend.

These noises are often heard at one of the routine examinations, or when there is an incidental infection. They are louder when the heart is beating faster than usual e.g. with a temperature, or if the child is particularly worried.

They are usually soft, heard in one area, change with sitting or lying, frequently have a buzzing or musical quality and are the only finding. The rest of the examination is normal.

The noise is often so typical that no tests are necessary. The family may be reassured that all is well and the child may be discharged with a normal heart and no restrictions.

VENTRICULAR SEPTAL DEFECT (VSD)

This is a hole between the two pumping chambers (ventricles). It allows some oxygenated blood to pass from the left side back into the right side and through the lungs. The amount of abnormal blood flow depends on the size and site of the hole as well as the pressure difference between the two sides of the heart. The abnormal flow produces the murmurs that are heard, and also the *thrill*, a vibration, which can be sometimes felt.

If the hole is small, the child is well and there are no problems. If the hole is moderate, the extra blood in the lungs makes them heavy and the child may breathe quickly, be slow to feed with poor weight gain, and have increased chest infections. These complaints are more marked if the hole is large.

The children with medium or large holes require medications, those with small ones do not. Echocardiography can show where it is, how big it is and often give an indication of whether it will close by itself.

Most holes will close spontaneously or get significantly smaller. Some will not and will require operation. The usual indications for operation are:

(i) *Failure to thrive adequately, despite medication in the first year of life.*

(ii) *The worry about high blood pressure in the lung arteries.*

(iii)*The persistence of a large blood flow into the lungs at over 7 years of age.*

(iv) *Development of a leaking aortic valve related to the hole.*

(v) *Development of extra muscle in the right ventricle secondary to the abnormal blood flow.*

The operation to close the hole, usually with a patch, is performed using the heart lung machine (cardiopulmonary bypass). Occasionally in small babies, or in those where there are additional significant problems, the blood flow to the lungs may be reduced by a preliminary operation – a banding, that narrows the lung artery.

Antibiotic prophylaxis is required, probably for one year after the spontaneous

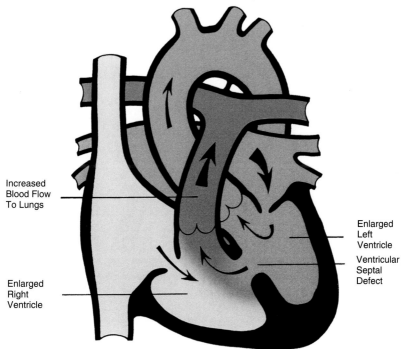

Increased Blood Flow To Lungs

Enlarged Left Ventricle

Ventricular Septal Defect

Enlarged Right Ventricle

VENTRICULAR SEPTAL DEFECT

closure of the hole. If the hole is closed surgically, and if there is no murmur and no residual leak, endocarditis prophylaxis can be stopped after one year.

If there is a residual murmur from a leak, or signs of leakage, antibiotics should be continued until these resolve.

ATRIAL SEPTAL DEFECT (ASD)

This is a hole between the two receiving chambers which allows blood from the left side to pass back to the right side and into the lungs.

There are three types: the commonest is in the middle of the atrial septum (the secundum defect). Sometimes it is in the lower part of the septum (the primum defect) and is associated with an abnormality (often a leak) of the mitral valve. Occasionally, it is in

the top of the septum (the sinus venosus defect) associated with an abnormality of the right upper lung vein.

Usually children have no symptoms, and a routine examination finds a murmur present. Occasionally, there is poor weight gain and failure to thrive.

Small defects that allow little blood to shunt from one side of the heart to the other often cause no problems. Such defects in the middle portion of the septum may close spontaneously in young children.

Moderate and large defects do not close by themselves, and the extra work which has to be done by the heart over many years into adult life causes a strain on its right side, with enlargement of the receiving chamber and pump chamber. As a result, the heart gets tired in middle life. The results of repairing the defect at that age

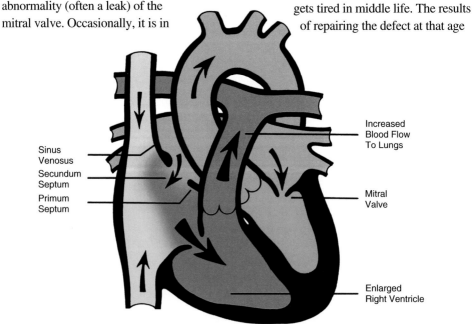

Sinus
Venosus

Secundum
Septum

Primum
Septum

Increased
Blood Flow
To Lungs

Mitral
Valve

Enlarged
Right Ventricle

SECUNDUM ATRIAL SEPTAL DEFECT

are not as good as when undertaken earlier. The plan, therefore is to close these defects during childhood.

Many which are in the mid portion of the atrial septum, have good margins, are free from adjacent structures and are not too large, can be closed by a plastic and metal device, or a plug inserted at cardiac catheterisation.

Aspirin is given for three months following this to reduce chances of clots developing on the device. Antibiotic prophylaxis is needed for only one year assuming the hole is closed.

In others, the defect will be too large or adjacent to important structures. This needs to be closed by open heart surgery either by direct suture or with a patch. Antibiotic prophylaxis is not required beyond a year after closure.

PARTIAL ATRIO-VENTRICULAR SEPTAL DEFECT

(Primum atrial septal defect)

This hole is at the bottom of the wall between two filling chambers and the defect also involves the valves between the filling chambers and the pumping chambers. The left sided valve may be very leaky and may cause early symptoms of breathlessness and poor weight gain.

This requires surgery. The hole is closed with a patch and the valve is usually repaired with sutures. Long-term follow-up is required and antibiotic prophylaxis is required for life.

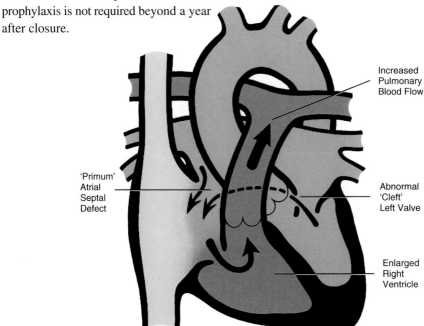

'Primum' Atrial Septal Defect

Increased Pulmonary Blood Flow

Abnormal 'Cleft' Left Valve

Enlarged Right Ventricle

PARTIAL ATRIO-VENTRICULAR SEPTAL DEFECT

page 19

PERSISTENT ARTERIAL DUCT
(Patent Ductus Arteriosus)

This is when the tube between the aorta and the lung artery, which is normally open when the baby is growing in the womb, fails to close after the birth as it should, i.e. it remains open – or "persistent".

It allows blood to pass from the high pressure aorta into the low pressure pulmonary artery and therefore increases the blood flow to the lungs. If the flow is small, there are no problems, if large the child will be breathless with tiredness and poor weight gain. It is common in premature babies.

If the tube (ductus) is still open more than three months, after the birth, it is unlikely to close on its own. Closure is advised in children with large tubes to reduce the workload on the heart and lungs and in small ones, to prevent the chance of infection developing in the tube (endarteritis). Many can now be closed by a catheter technique using either coils or plugs. Antibiotic prophylaxis is required for a year after implantation, then if there is no leak, may be stopped.

If the tube is large and the child small, surgical closure is often the best solution. The operation is performed through the left side of the chest without needing a heart lung machine and the tube is tied, clipped or divided. This can sometimes be performed with minimal invasive surgery (thorascopically). Circulation then returns to normal. The child may usually be discharged from follow-up with a normal heart. Antibiotic prophylaxis is then no longer required.

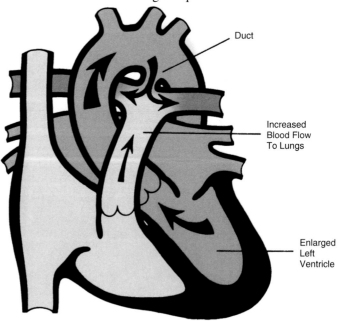

Duct

Increased
Blood Flow
To Lungs

Enlarged
Left
Ventricle

PERSISTENT ARTERIAL DUCT

COARCTATION OF THE AORTA

This is a narrowing in the main artery to the body usually just below the origin of the left arm artery. It may be associated with abnormalities of the ventricular septum, aortic and mitral valves. The narrowing increases the work on the left ventricle, raises the pressure in the top half of the body, and reduces it in the lower half. If severe, it can present early in life with breathlessness, difficulty in feeding and occasionally, very rapid deterioration in the baby's health. More moderate obstruction produces a murmur, high blood pressure, and weak pulses in the legs. With mild obstruction, a soft murmur is often picked up at school, and examination reveals weak pulses in the legs.

If the child has symptoms or high blood pressure, operation to relieve the obstruction is necessary at that stage. If the obstruction is very mild, regular review in Out-patients is necessary. The operation is carried out through the left chest, without using the heart/lung machine. The narrow area can be directly removed, occasionally it is patched with artificial material or the first part of the left arm artery may be used to effect the repair.

Long term follow-up is necessary to check on blood pressure and for any evidence of re-narrowing. This re-narrowing is more likely to occur if the operation is performed during the first few months of life. If this happens, then balloon stretching of a narrow area with a catheter test may be necessary or very occasionally, further re-operation.

Some centres have recently been stretching initial coarctation with balloon catheters in older children and in young adults, ballooning and stenting of the narrow area has been used with very encouraging early results.

Antibiotic prophylaxis is required long term as coarctation is frequently associated with aortic and mitral valve problems.

Coarctation

Thick Left Ventricle

COARCTATION OF THE AORTA

AORTIC STENOSIS

This is a narrowing between the left ventricle and the aorta. The commonest is valvar stenosis where the leaflets which are normally thin become thick and have restricted opening. This increases the work of the left ventricle. Severity is variable and even very significant obstruction can cause no symptoms. Complaints of fainting and breathlessness may occur and need assessment. Moderate and severe obstruction require avoidance of competitive sport, rowing, judo and karate. ECG and echo Doppler are very helpful in assessing severity and monitoring change.

Relief of obstruction is required for significant stenosis. The options vary between different hospitals. Some will offer balloon dilatation with a catheter technique as the first treatment, others will offer surgery using the heart lung machine. There is clearly no answer that suits every patient. If a balloon technique is used, we would expect to be able to lessen the obstruction.

Occasionally no benefit happens and other times, the valve leaks significantly afterwards.

If the operation is chosen, this is open heart surgery using a heart lung machine. The valve is inspected, stretched and often thinned. Very occasionally, it would need to be replaced at the first operation. Either surgical stretching – or balloon stretching – improves the valve but it is likely to thicken again over the years ahead, requiring long-term follow-up, and probably, further procedures.

With subvalvar aortic stenosis, a 'shelf' occurs between the left ventricle and the aortic valve. This requires 'open heart' surgery to remove it when the obstruction is severe. With supravalvar stenosis there is a waist above the aortic valve and above the coronary arteries. If the obstruction is severe then this needs to be patched, again using 'open heart' surgery. Antibiotic prophylaxis is required lifelong in all these children.

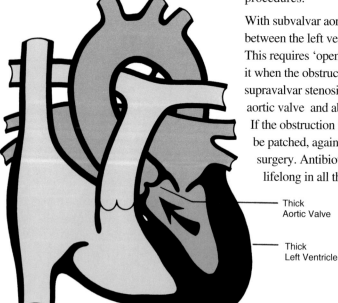

Thick
Aortic Valve

Thick
Left Ventricle

AORTIC VALVE STENOSIS

PULMONARY STENOSIS

The pulmonary valve leaflets are thickened and have restricted opening. The right ventricle has extra work to do and becomes thicker. If the valve is very tight, blueness will present early in life. If the obstruction is moderate, a murmur will be picked up at routine examination.

Mild obstruction is tolerated very well over a long period of time. Moderate and severe obstruction requires relief. The valve can be stretched and this is usually performed by a balloon catheter. Generally, the results of ballooning these valves have been very good. In some cases the ballooning procedure is not possible, particularly in small babies where the obstruction is very severe, and in some older children whose valves are very thick. This may be associated with Noonan's syndrome. In these cases, an operation to stretch or remove the valve, would be required. The long term outlook is good. Mild leaking is well tolerated. Antibiotic prophylaxis requirement is being debated.

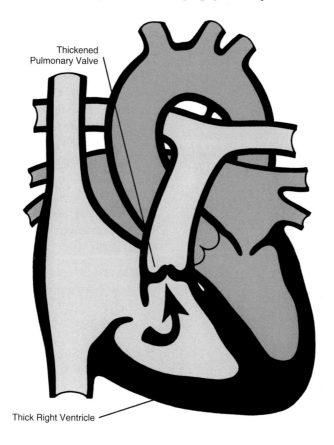

Thickened Pulmonary Valve

Thick Right Ventricle

PULMONARY VALVE STENOSIS

page 23

TETRALOGY OF FALLOT

This is a combination of a hole between the two ventricles, and a narrowing between the right ventricle and the lung artery. The right ventricle has extra work to do to squeeze blood through the narrowing to the lungs, and as it works at high pressure, is able to pump blood directly from it through the intraventricular hole into the aorta.

A murmur may be noted initially and then blueness and perhaps squatting will occur during the second year. If the problem is more severe, then blueness will present earlier.

Some children have 'spells' in which the blood flow to the lungs is reduced for a while. The child may cry abnormally as though in discomfort, breathe quickly, become bluer than usual and perhaps have glazed eyes, whimper and then become rather limp, pale and then pass off to sleep. If these episodes occur, picking the child up and cuddling and reassuring is very helpful. Put the child over your shoulder bringing the knees up onto his tummy, so that they are between his tummy and your chest. This improves the circulation and the episode will subside. It is important to let the medical team involved, know that these 'spells' have started to occur. Propranolol, a medicine, can help reduce these episodes. All children will require operation in due course.

In many, open heart surgical repair to patch the hole and relieve the narrowing which may require a patch across the pulmonary valve can be undertaken directly. In others, particularly if the child is small or the lung arteries are small, then a shunt operation to take extra blood into the lung arteries from an arm artery may be required (see page 27). This operation is performed either through the side of the chest, or the breastbone (sternum) and a formal repair would be planned for later.

The long term results are usually very good. Sometimes, a further operation is required in those who have a significant leak of blood back from the lung artery into the right sided chamber. This is more likely in those who required a large patch across the pulmonary valve at the time of their operation. A new biological pulmonary valve will be inserted which improves symptoms and the efficiency of the circulation.

Long-term follow-up and antibiotic prophylaxis is required.

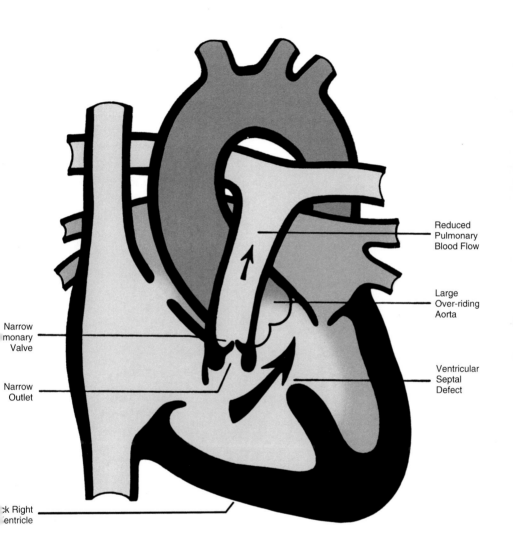

Reduced
Pulmonary
Blood Flow

Large
Over-riding
Aorta

Narrow
monary
Valve

Narrow
Outlet

Ventricular
Septal
Defect

ck Right
entricle

TETRALOGY OF FALLOT

page 25

TRICUSPID ATRESIA

The tricuspid valve is absent and the right ventricle is usually small. There is usually a reduced blood flow to the lungs.

Blood has to pass from the right atrium into the left atrium, then into the left ventricle from which most of the blood will go to the body. Some blood will go through a hole in the ventricular septum into the small right ventricle and then into the lungs. These children usually present with blueness and murmurs early on in life, and occasionally 'spells' like tetralogy of Fallot.

Increasing the blood flow to the lungs is necessary by a shunt procedure when symptoms warrant. In small babies, this is likely to be an arterial shunt connecting one of the arm arteries to the lung artery. In older infants and young children, a venous shunt can be created joining the upper body vein (the superior vena cava) directly into the lung artery (a Glenn shunt – see diagram, page 37).

Definitive surgery involves directing blood returning to the heart from the body directly into the lung artery. Initially, this involved connecting the right atrium to the lung arteries and closing the hole between the filling chambers. This is the Fontan procedure. Over the years, there have been many modifications of this operation

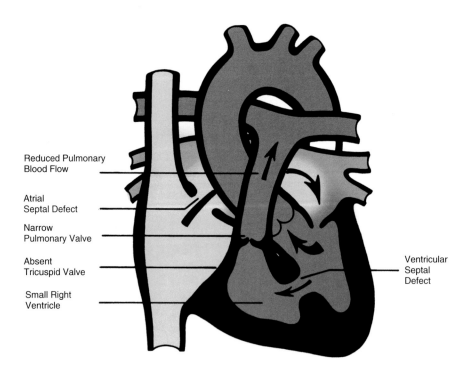

Reduced Pulmonary
Blood Flow

Atrial
Septal Defect

Narrow
Pulmonary Valve

Absent
Tricuspid Valve

Small Right
Ventricle

Ventricular
Septal
Defect

TRICUSPID ATRESIA

improving the pattern of blood flow from the veins into the lung artery (total cavopulmonary connection).

For these operations to be successful, they require good size lung arteries with low pressures within them, a good functioning left ventricle (main pump chamber) with no leaking of the mitral valve.

This is a big operation. The recovery period is slower than for many other forms of cardiac surgery. Chest drains frequently need to be left in for a week or two as the body gets used to having high pressures within the veins. There is gradual and continued improvement in well being over many months after discharge. Medicines are usually required also for many months, some units thinning the blood with Aspirin, others formally anti-coagulate the patient long-term with Warfarin.

Often a small communication (called a 'fenestration' or 'window') is created in the wall between the flow pattern to the lungs and the left filling chamber (left atrium). This acts as a 'safety valve' and allows some blood to short circuit the lungs. It is useful in the early postoperative course and often gets spontaneously smaller with time. However, if a significant flow of blue blood into the other side of the heart persists, then this fenestration can be plugged later with a catheter technique.

Children frequently remain with a high colour and blue hands and feet and remain a little tired on strenuous exercise. Most however, are able to play games at school and enjoy normal activities. In some children, further operations to improve and streamline blood flow into the heart are necessary. Irregularities of heart rhythm requiring long term medications may occur in young adult life. Antibiotic prophylaxis and long-term follow-up is required.

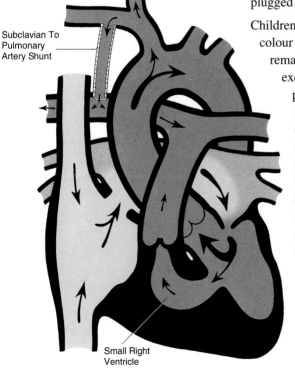

Subclavian To Pulmonary Artery Shunt

Small Right Ventricle

SUBCLAVIAN TO PULMONARY ARTERY SHUNT

PULMONARY ATRESIA WITH NO VENTRICULAR SEPTAL DEFECT

In pulmonary atresia with an intact ventricular septum, the pulmonary valve is blocked and blood flow to the lungs depends on whether the pre-birth arterial duct remains open. The right ventricle is of variable size and may be small.

If it is very small, it is unlikely to grow and a shunt procedure alone is necessary to take extra blood into the lungs aiming for a Fontan type operation in due course. If the right ventricle is larger, then the pulmonary valve may be stretched or removed and a shunt procedure is usually undertaken at the same time. Sometimes, by using a catheter technique, it is possible to cross this blocked valve with a special wire and then stretch the valve with a balloon, allowing blood to go from the heart directly towards the lung artery. Additionally, a shunt operation would often need to be performed, but this can be done with closed heart surgery.

Further operations are usually necessary to relieve residual obstruction or to overcome leaking in the area of the pulmonary valve. In some, the right ventricle is of a good size, the shunt can be closed and the hole between the filling chambers closed. In others, the upper body vein can be joined to the lung artery reducing some of the work of the right ventricle and in others, a Fontan type operation is the best long term plan.

Long term follow-up and antibiotic prophylaxis is necessary.

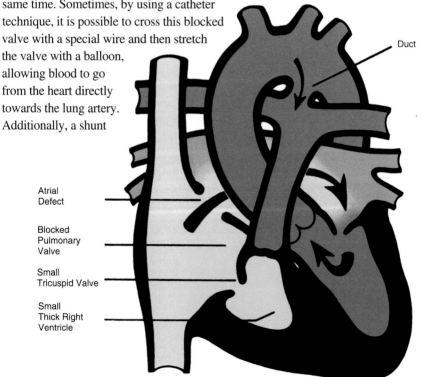

Duct

Atrial Defect

Blocked Pulmonary Valve

Small Tricuspid Valve

Small Thick Right Ventricle

PULMONARY ATRESIA WITH NO VENTRICULAR SEPTAL DEFECT

PULMONARY ATRESIA WITH VENTRICULAR SEPTAL DEFECT

There is complete blockage between the heart and the lung arteries, and a hole between the two pumping chambers. The right ventricle is of good size in this condition. Blood supply to the lungs may be from the duct or from collateral vessels.

Detailed angiographic studies are required to look at the collateral vessels and lung circulation in order to plan the optimum management for each child. Many will require shunt procedures to increase the blood flow to the lungs. These shunts may be performed through the side of the chest or through the breast bone.

Often, the lung arteries are very small, and a series of shunts may be necessary joining up the central lung arteries to a number of the extra collateral vessels *(unifocalisation)*. The hope is to produce an adequate sized source of blood supply to each lung which can in due course be connected to the right pump chamber.

In some patients, the collateral vessels themselves can be stretched with balloons and stented via a catheter technique to improve the blood flow towards the lung. In other patients, no operation or procedure is required as the condition is reasonably well balanced.

Chromosome tests are often performed. Long term follow-up and antibiotic prophylaxis is required.

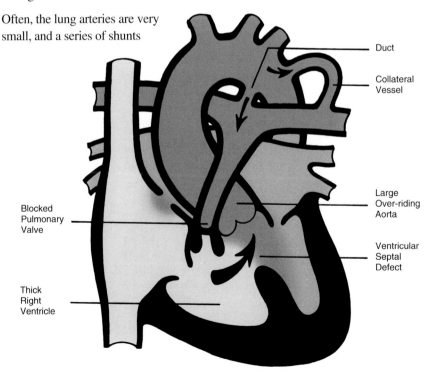

Duct

Collateral Vessel

Large Over-riding Aorta

Ventricular Septal Defect

Blocked Pulmonary Valve

Thick Right Ventricle

PULMONARY ATRESIA WITH VENTRICULAR SEPTAL DEFECT

SIMPLE TRANSPOSITION

The aorta rises from the right ventricle, and the pulmonary artery from the left ventricle. Blue, relatively deoxygenated blood is thus directed back to the body and pink oxygenated blood from the lungs is directed back into the lungs.

These children present early in life with 'blueness' (cyanosis). Usually a hole is made between the two receiving chambers of the heart using a procedure with a special catheter – *a balloon septostomy*, allowing the two blood streams to mix.

The operation which is now preferred is an 'arterial switch' to put the arteries back onto their normal ventricles, at the same time re-implanting the coronary arteries. This needs to be carried out in the first weeks of life while the left ventricle is still relatively thick walled. It is a large, open heart operation. Occasionally, a different operation redirecting the blood flow throughout the atrium, the Senning or Mustard procedure, is advised and this may be deferred until later in the first year of life. These were the operations that were most commonly performed until the late 1980s. In them, the left ventricle continues to pump blood to the lungs with the right ventricle pumping to the body.

The majority of children with both types of operation are very well afterwards and enjoy all normal activities.

Long-term follow-up is required and possibly antibiotic prophylaxis, but if the circulations are working well, it may not be necessary.

Aorta

Pulmonary Artery

Atrial Septal Defect

Left Ventricle

Right Ventricle

SIMPLE TRANSPOSITION OF GREAT ARTERIES

COMPLEX TRANSPOSITION

*1) Transposition with
   ventricular septal defect.*
*2) Transposition with
   persistent arterial duct.*

In both these conditions, there is a large communication between the two separate circulations.

Despite this, most centres would advise making an additional hole between the two receiving chambers (balloon septostomy) by a catheter. The children are frequently only moderately blue but very breathless. They need medications to support their heart and require early surgery. Repair involves switching the arteries back to normal, re-implanting the coronary arteries and closing the communication. This is a large operation requiring open heart surgery and is usually undertaken in the first weeks of life to prevent damage occurring to the lung arteries. Occasionally, banding or narrowing is put on the lung artery if the communication is particularly difficult to close, and open surgery thus delayed.

*3) Transposition with ventricular septal
   defect and pulmonary stenosis.*

The lungs are protected by the narrowing between the heart and the lung artery. The hole between the two pumping chambers

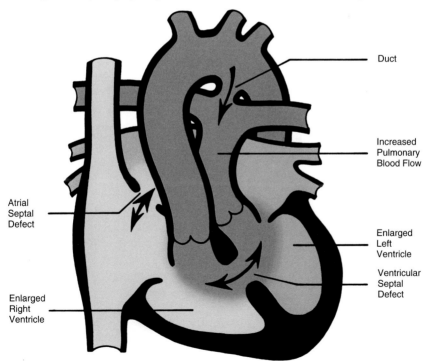

Duct

Increased
Pulmonary
Blood Flow

Atrial
Septal
Defect

Enlarged
Left
Ventricle

Ventricular
Septal
Defect

Enlarged
Right
Ventricle

**TRANSPOSITION WITH VENTRICULAR SEPTAL DEFECT
PERSISTENT DUCT AND ATRIAL SEPTAL DEFECT**

allows the two streams of blood to mix, and therefore, these children are not as blue as those with simple transposition. However, as the months go by, the obstruction to blood flow increases, and a shunt procedure and enlarging of the atrial hole is frequently required.

The obstruction between the heart and the lung arteries is difficult to relieve directly and usually has to be bypassed by a valved artificial tube (a conduit) placed between the right ventricle and the lung artery. The hole between the pumping chambers is closed so that the left pump chamber directs blood into the aorta. This operation is often postponed until the children are four to six years of age to allow an adequate sized tube to be inserted.

This is a major operation requiring open heart surgery, and is often referred to as a Rastelli procedure. As the tubes implanted at the operation do not allow for growth, they get relatively narrower and often need replacing in later life.

Long term follow-up and antibiotic prophylaxis is required.

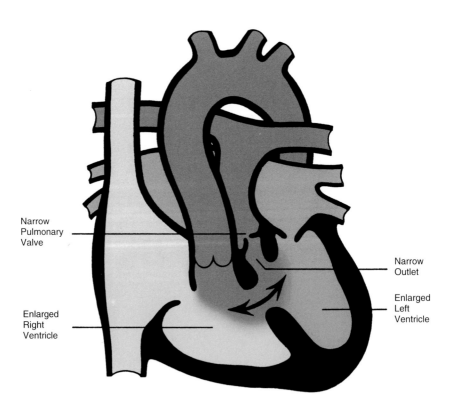

Narrow Pulmonary Valve

Narrow Outlet

Enlarged Left Ventricle

Enlarged Right Ventricle

TRANSPOSITION WITH VENTRICULAR SEPTAL DEFECT AND PULMONARY STENOSIS

COMPLETE ATRIO-VENTRICULAR SEPTAL DEFECT

There is a large hole in the wall between all four chambers of the heart – and only one single valve between them in the middle of the heart.

The hole allows excess blood to pass from the left to the right side of the heart. If the valve leaks, this further increases the work of the heart by allowing blood to be pumped backwards into the receiving chambers as well as forwards into the arteries.

Repair is usually planned early in life before damage to the lung arteries occurs. The holes between the filling chambers and the pump chambers are closed with patches and the single valve is divided into halves, the middle portions of the valve being attached to the patch. In some babies, narrowing of the lung artery (a banding) may be performed in the first instance to protect the lungs and allow very small children to grow. The majority of children are significantly improved as a result of their surgery. Residual leaking of repaired valves can be a problem and if severe, further surgery may be necessary. Long-term follow-up and antibiotic prophylaxis is required.

This is one of the commonest heart problems occurring in Down's syndrome.

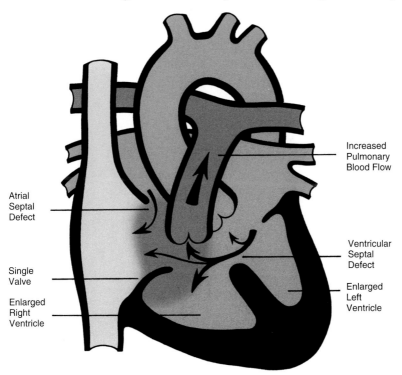

Atrial Septal Defect

Single Valve

Enlarged Right Ventricle

Increased Pulmonary Blood Flow

Ventricular Septal Defect

Enlarged Left Ventricle

COMPLETE ATRIO-VENTRICULAR SEPTAL DEFECT

ANOMALOUS PULMONARY VENOUS CONNECTION

The pulmonary veins, instead of connecting into the left atrium, connect into the right side of the circulation. If only *some* of the veins drain (connect) abnormally, the term *'partial'* is used. If *all* the connections drain abnormally, the condition is decribed as *'total'*.

There are several sites into which the veins may drain. These are shown in the diagram and may be above the heart into the large veins (1 or 2), within the heart either into the right atrium or coronary sinus (3 or 4); or below the heart into the liver or into the major lower vein (5).

If the connection is narrow (obstructed) then the child will present in the early days of life with blueness and breathlessness because blood has difficulty in returning from the lungs into the heart. If the connection is wide open (non-obstructed) then the problems are breathlessness, chest infections and poor weight gain and

come to light during the first months of life rather than the first few days.

Open heart surgery to redirect the blood flow back into the left atrium is required when symptoms (complaints) occur. Although the operation is complex and initial recovery slow, particularly in those where the connection is obstructed, the long term outlook is often good. Occasionally, further obstruction occurs with growth which may be at the new connection into the heart or within the lung veins themselves. Long-term follow-up is required but long term antibiotic prophylaxis is not necessary beyond a year after the operation.

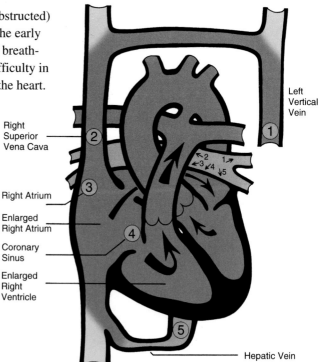

Left Vertical Vein

Right Superior Vena Cava

Right Atrium

Enlarged Right Atrium

Coronary Sinus

Enlarged Right Ventricle

Hepatic Vein

TOTAL ANOMALOUS PULMONARY VENOUS DRAINAGE

DOUBLE INLET VENTRICLE

In this group of conditions there is a large pumping chamber (ventricle) into which both atria empty their blood through either one or two valves. There is usually a second smaller pump chamber at the side of the main ventricle. The arteries commonly come one from each ventricle as in the diagram or both may arise from one of the ventricles.

If there is no additional narrowing to the flow of blood into the lungs, the child will be breathless, feed poorly and gain weight slowly. Often narrowing, or banding, of the lung artery will be required in the first instance. If there is severe obstruction of blood flow to the lungs, then the child will be blue and may require the blood supply to the lungs to be increased with a shunt operation.

If there is narrowing between the main pump chamber and the body artery, either within the heart or in the aorta (coarctation), then this obstruction needs to be relieved and the vessels to the lungs protected. This is a much more complex and serious problem.

In some children, the circulation is very nicely balanced, not too breathless, nor too blue and steady progress is made. However, most need help and can be improved by these initial operations with a view to later planning a Fontan-type operation connecting the large veins to the body directly to the lung artery and leaving the main ventricle and smaller ventricle pumping blood to the body.

Long-term follow-up and antibiotic prophylaxis is required.

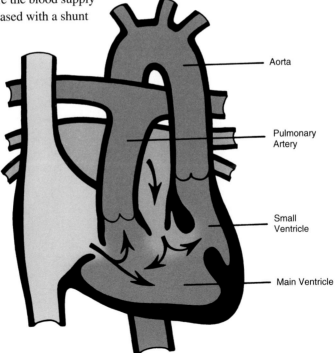

Aorta

Pulmonary Artery

Small Ventricle

Main Ventricle

DOUBLE INLET VENTRICLE

HYPOPLASTIC LEFT HEART SYNDROME

The main pumping chamber (the left ventricle) is very small and the aortic and mitral valves are either very narrow, thickened, or entirely blocked.

The babies are in major difficulties in the first few days of life as changes in the circulation occur with closure of the duct. This is one of the most serious of all heart abnormalities and remains a very difficult area despite the advances that have been made in general over the years.

Early open heart surgery is often recommended. This involves joining the small aorta to the start of the large lung artery and dividing this from the branches of the lung artery which are then connected with a shunt from the innominate artery. Arch obstruction (co-arctation) is patched and in addition, the hole between the receiving chambers is enlarged.

This remains a very big operation and leaves the right ventricle pumping blood to the body and also to the lungs via the shunt. This is called a Norwood Stage I operation (see illustration on the right).

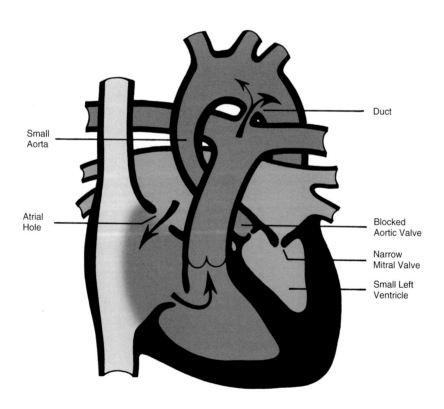

Small Aorta

Duct

Atrial Hole

Blocked Aortic Valve

Narrow Mitral Valve

Small Left Ventricle

HYPOPLASTIC LEFT HEART SYNDROME

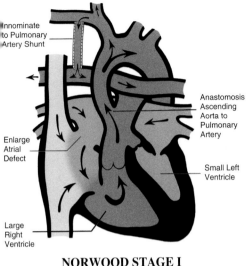

Innominate to Pulmonary Artery Shunt

Anastomosis Ascending Aorta to Pulmonary Artery

Enlarge Atrial Defect

Small Left Ventricle

Large Right Ventricle

NORWOOD STAGE I

Later, following a catheter test, the upper body vein (the superior vena cava) is joined to the right lung artery. This is called a Norwood Stage II operation – or a Glenn shunt. (see illustration below left).

Later again, at perhaps 2-4 years of age depending on clinical progress and after a further catheter test, the lower body vein is joined to the lung artery with a further operation known as Norwood Stage III.

This produces Fontan-type circulation (total cavo-pulmonary connection).

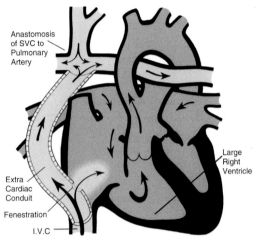

Anastomosis of SVC to Pulmonary Artery

Large Right Ventricle

Extra Cardiac Conduit

Fenestration

I.V.C

NORWOOD STAGE III

The children require close follow-up, and feeding difficulties are very common in the first months of life. Some children, because of problems with lung arteries or heart muscle function, may be considered for heart transplantion in due course.

This congenital heart disorder remains a very difficult area and there is a need for a very wide discussion with the family in the early days. Long-term follow-up and antibiotic prophylaxis is required.

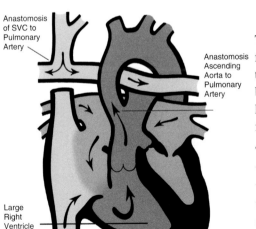

Anastomosis of SVC to Pulmonary Artery

Anastomosis Ascending Aorta to Pulmonary Artery

Large Right Ventricle

NORWOOD STAGE II

COMMON ARTERIAL TRUNK

(Truncus Arteriosus)

There is one large single artery arising from the heart which then divides into the lung artery and the body artery. There is, in addition, a large hole between the two pumping chambers.

This problem allows a very high blood flow to the lung, which makes the child breathless, liable to repeated infections, and to gain weight poorly.

Initial help is given with medicines, but an operation to repair the problem is necessary within the first weeks of life.

This involves closing the hole between the pumping chambers, and taking the lung artery off the side of the body artery, connecting it with a conduit (a tube) to the right ventricle. The operation needs to be performed before the lung arteries are damaged by the high flow and a high pressure.

This is a large operation and in due course, the conduit will need to be replaced as the child grows.

Chromosome tests are often performed. Long-term follow-up and antibiotic prophylaxis is required.

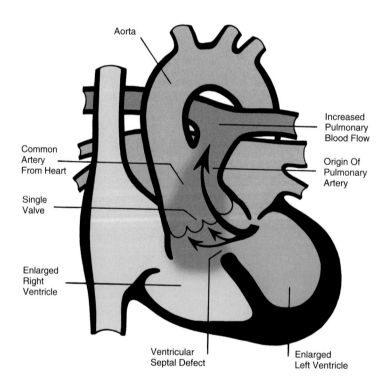

Aorta

Increased Pulmonary Blood Flow

Common Artery From Heart

Origin Of Pulmonary Artery

Single Valve

Enlarged Right Ventricle

Ventricular Septal Defect

Enlarged Left Ventricle

COMMON ARTERIAL TRUNK

DILATED CARDIOMYOPATHY

In this condition the muscle of the heart is weak and the heart usually enlarged.

Young children present with feeding difficulties, breathlessness, poor weight gain and recurrent chest infections.

Older children and adolescents present with tiredness, weakness, breathlessness and weight loss. The cause in many is unknown. In some, it may be related to previous viral infections. In others, there may be a genetic predisposition.

Several medicines are often required long term to make the heart work more efficiently e.g. Ace inhibitors, Digoxin, beta blockers. Others remove excess fluid e.g. diuretics and others are used to thin blood to reduce the chance of clots developing within the circulation e.g. Aspirin or Warfarin. Not all children need all these medicines.

Many children gradually improve. In some, the damage to the heart muscle is more severe and their condition gets worse. If this happens, despite large doses of many medicines, heart transplantation may be considered.

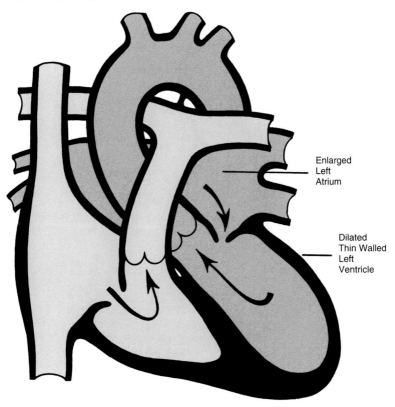

Enlarged Left Atrium

Dilated Thin Walled Left Ventricle

DILATED CARDIOMYOPATHY

HYPERTROPHIC CARDIOMYOPATHY

In this condition, the heart muscle is very thick and has difficulty in relaxing. Sometimes the extra muscle causes obstruction to blood flow out of the heart.

Many cases are mild with no symptoms, others have dizziness, fainting attacks, palpitations and chest discomfort. There may be other family members who are affected by this condition.

Regular drugs are used if symptoms are present and these help improve relaxation of the heart muscle and control abnormalities of heart rhythm. If the obstruction is severe an operation to remove some of the excess muscle may be performed. Long-term follow-up and antibiotic prophylaxis is necessary.

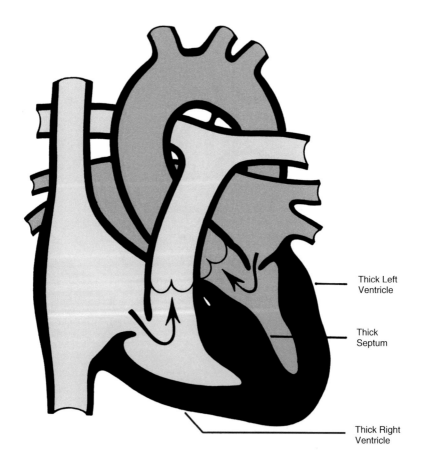

Thick Left Ventricle

Thick Septum

Thick Right Ventricle

HYPERTROPHIC CARDIOMYOPATHY

page 40

PULMONARY HYPERTENSION OF THE NEWBORN

(Persistent fetal circulation)

The heart and lungs themselves are formed normally, but the lung arteries in both lungs remain narrow and constricted as they are in the womb.

As a result of this, the pressure in the lung artery remains very high and de-oxygenated blood is directed across the small flap valve between the atria and also across the duct between the arteries.

It is often difficult to differentiate this condition from structural heart problems and babies are thus often referred to Cardiac Units.

The management of this condition consists of ventilation and medicines e.g. nitric oxide, prostaglandin, to open up the lung arteries.

In others, the arteries do not open up and the child's condition can be very critical. Use of a special heart lung machine known as ECMO (Extracorporeal Membrane Oxygenation) may be required. (see page 57 for details)

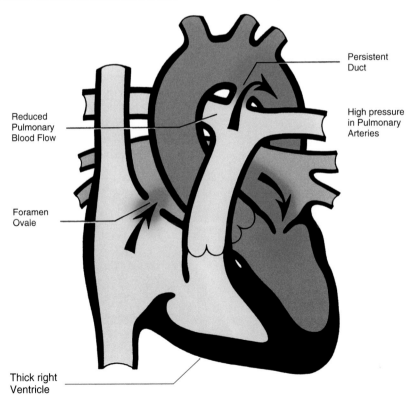

Persistent Duct

High pressure in Pulmonary Arteries

Reduced Pulmonary Blood Flow

Foramen Ovale

Thick right Ventricle

PERSISTENT FETAL CIRCULATION

4 INTERVENTIONAL CATHETERISATION

About balloons, blades, stents, plugs & coils

An increasing number of conditions can now be treated in the Catheter Laboratory, thus avoiding formal operations. The first procedures performed were the use of the inflatable balloon catheter to enlarge the

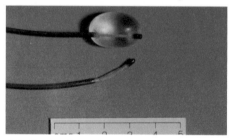

A balloon catheter for transposition.

small hole in the wall between the two filling chambers *(the septum)* of the heart, in new born babies with transposition of the great arteries *(see page 30)*.

This revolutionised the care of these babies by allowing the two separate streams of blood to mix, thus enabling a better oxygen supply to the body. In older children with various heart problems, a hole can also be made in this wall *(the septum)* and then enlarged with an expandable blade and balloon to improve the mixing of blood.

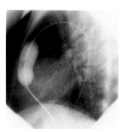

X-ray picture of a balloon catheter dilating a pulmonary valve

Narrowing (stenosis) of the pulmonary, aortic, and occasionally rheumatic mitral valves, can be stretched with expandable balloons by placing them temporarily across the narrow valve. Ballooning the valve relieves the obstruction, but may produce some degree of leakage afterwards. This is not important with the pulmonary valve, but may be so, with the aortic or mitral valves.

Arteries can also be dilated or made wider (often following previous surgery) for example: pulmonary arterial stenosis following tetralogy of Fallot repair, or re-coarctation of the aorta. Sometimes the arteries are elastic and recoil when the balloon is deflated. They then need to be re-stretched and held open with a device called a balloon-expandable stent (a wire cage – see below).

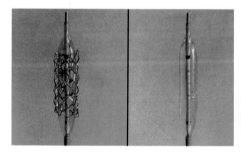

A balloon catheter (right) fitted with an expandable wire stent (left) which will be inserted into a blood vessel to prevent it from narrowing again.

Abnormal blood vessels can be blocked with coils or plugs, for example, in conditions such as persistent arterial duct or collateral vessels.

Atrial septal defects, when the hole is in the middle portion of the wall between the two filling chambers, with good distances from surrounding veins and valves, may be closed with various plugs. Occasionally, holes in the middle or lower portion of the wall between the two ventricles (muscular ventricular septum), can also be plugged by different shaped devices. (picture below).

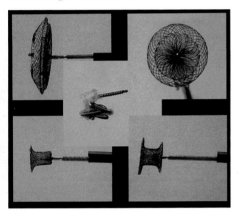

Different devices which can be delivered with the catheter to close holes and vessels.

The latest development that looks to be very promising, is the placement of an expandable artificial valve in the lung artery position for patients with significant pulmonary regurgitation (leakage).

These devices or plugs are usually made of a special type of wire that has a 'memory' of its original shape. They can be collapsed down into a fine delivery catheter. The catheter can be placed across the defect and then with either, or both X-ray and ultrasound control (often with transoesophageal echocardiography), the device can be delivered to the appropriate position, where it returns to its original shape, blocking the abnormality. Very occasionally these plugs can move and may need to be retrieved, either with a further catheter technique, or occasionally via an operation.

Most of the procedures described here in this chapter are performed under general anaesthesia and the patient can be discharged, usually within 24 hours.

Antibiotic prophylaxis is usually required long-term when arteries are stretched and for a year after complete and successful closures of holes or abnormal vessels.

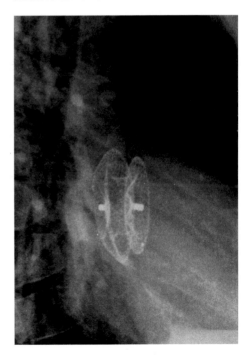

X-ray picture showing an expandable wire A.S.D. device positioned in the heart.

5 ARRHYTHMIAS & PACEMAKERS

The heart has its own complex electrical system. It can have a primary fault in an otherwise normal heart, or may be abnormal as a result of a congenital or acquired heart disease, or operation.

The specialised cells which are grouped at the junction of the superior vena cava and the right atrium are called the sinus node and have the fastest rate of activation and recovery of all normal heart cells. They thus control the normal heart rhythm. They have an abundant supply of nerves which can speed up the heart (sympathetic) or slow it down (parasympathetic/vagus). The electrical activity from the sinus node spreads out over the atrium

causing the atria to contract. The signal then passes into a "junction box" which is called the *atrio-ventricular node* in the floor of the right atrium. There is a pause of about one to two-tenths of a second and then the signal runs rapidly in the only connection to the pump chamber via the fast conducting system *(Bundle of His and Purkinje fibres)*. This spreads the activity to

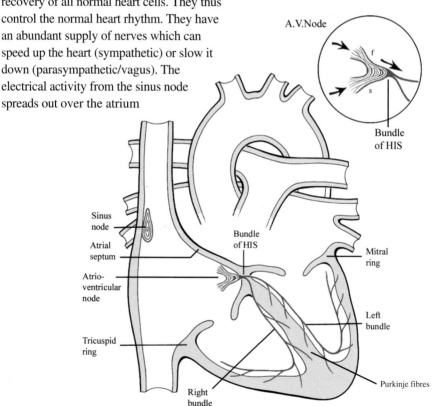

NORMAL ELECTRIC CIRCUIT

all parts of the ventricles causing them to contract in a synchronised way. Following this, the cells recover (called *repolarisation*), the muscles relax and then the process starts over again with the *sinus node* cells recovering the fastest. The atrium and ventricles are insulated from each other by fibrous and fatty tissue and the only normal way through is the *Bundle of His*.

Extra beats interposed between normal beats are very common and they produce extra 'thumps'. These are *benign* (harmless) and reassurance is all that is necessary.

Arrhythmia is a general term for an abnormal heart rhythm. It may occur as an isolated problem where the heart is otherwise normal, or in addition to an underlying structural problem.

Bradycardia

This is when the heart rate is relatively slow, rather like that of an athlete. Often there are no symptoms. If the heart rate becomes too low to meet the usual demands, the child may complain of dizziness, light-headedness, tiredness and breathlessness. The problem maybe that the heart's natural pacemaker *(the sinus node)* is too slow, or that there is a problem within the heart's "junction box" *(the atrio-ventricular node)* that does not allow the normal conduction of the impulses from the top chamber to the bottom chamber. This is termed 'heart block'. With this, the bottom chambers' spontaneous rate is often very slow. If the symptoms occur and are confirmed by tests, such as ECG/24 hour tape/event recorder,

then the heart's action needs to be speeded up. This is usually performed with a pacemaker. This problem can occur if the heart is otherwise normal or in association with a congenital heart disease, either before or after operations.

A pacemaker consists of a battery and a complex electronic circuit which controls its power and speed. Advances in electronics mean that pacemakers are now much smaller then before. Current models are less than the size of a matchbox weighing around about 50 - 60 grams *(see pictures on page 46)*. The battery can be implanted under the skin and connected by one or two fine wires, either to the outside of the heart *(the epicardium – see pictures on page 46)* or to the inside of the heart (the endocardium) using a vein. With the epicardial type, the wire is sewn on to the

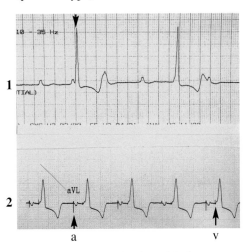

Upper trace 1: Complete heart block (slow ventricular rate).

Lower trace 2: Pacing spikes (arrowed) from implanted pacemaker precede atrial (a) and ventricular (v) signals.

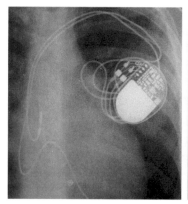

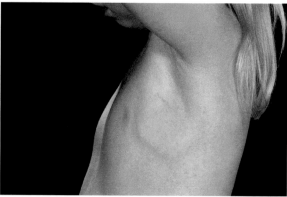

X-ray picture of a pacemaker

Site of a pacemaker

outside of the heart during an operation. The endocardial pacemaker has its fine wires inserted through a vein and steered into the heart under X-ray control in a catheter laboratory. *(see pictures on page 49).*

The decision of which type of pacemaker to use will depend on the age of the child and the underlying heart problem.

All pacemakers are now programmable, that is, their rate, power supply and timing can be

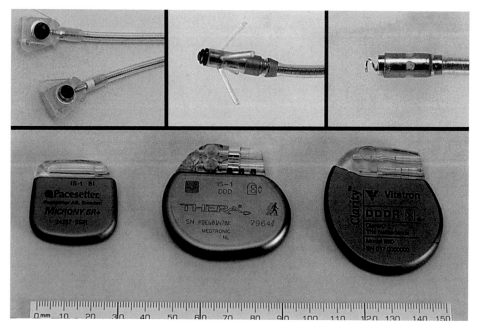

Three types of artificial pacemakers. The largest is only 40mm wide.
The top row picture shows the leads which are actually attached to the heart.

altered externally after the pacemaker has been inserted. This is done with a 'programmer' that sends signals from outside the body and can be done in outpatients. These alterations allow the settings to be finely adjusted for each individual child to maximise the efficiency of the system and the life of the battery. Most of the new pacemakers are termed 'physiological', which means that they can alter the rate of the heart pacing in response to exercise and emotion.

The majority of pacing systems now being inserted are expected to last 6 to 8 years. At that time the pacing box containing its batteries would need to be removed and replaced with a new one. Hopefully, the wire connecting the battery to the heart would not need to be replaced. However, with growth, the leads may become too short and too tight and may need to be removed and a new lead inserted. This is undertaken in the catheter room and can sometimes be a difficult procedure.

Regular follow-up to check the pacemaker is operating correctly will be required but this is not too frequent. Antibiotic prophylaxis is not necessary if the heart is otherwise normal.

Very little interference from outside electrical sources is likely, but being close to strong electrical fields such as those with 'dodgem' cars at the fairground or electric arc welding should be avoided. Most occupations and activities can be undertaken. Ordinary driving licences may be held, but not those for heavy goods vehicles or passenger vehicles.

Tachycardia

This occurs when the heart rate is abnormally fast for the needs of the body. It can occur in an otherwise normal heart or may be as a result of a congenital heart problem or related to previous surgery. Many of the tachycardias occur as a result of a re-entry circuit occurring within the heart. Different parts of the heart have different properties of conduction and recovery. The extra beats that happen in everyone can highlight these differences, allowing conduction to be blocked in one of these areas, whilst going down the other way and re-echoing back up the previously blocked area and then quickly down the first path again. This completes the circuit. Each time the electrical signal goes down into the pump chamber, the pump chamber

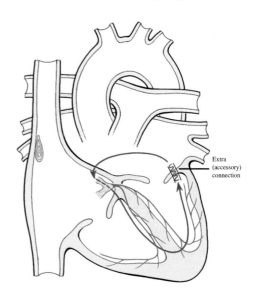

Extra
(accessory)
connection

**ATRIO-VENTRICULAR
RE-ENTRY CIRCUIT**

contracts and this produces the heart beat and the palpitation if the rate is fast.

The commonest condition of this type in young children is when there is an abnormal extra connection between the atrium and the ventricles across the insulating area. This is called *atrio-ventricular re-entry tachycardia*.

This may show an abnormal pattern on the ECG called pre-excitation *(Wolff-Parkinson White syndrome)*, but often does not (termed *'concealed'*).

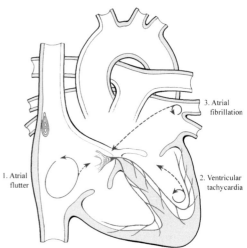

3. Atrial fibrillation

1. Atrial flutter

2. Ventricular tachycardia

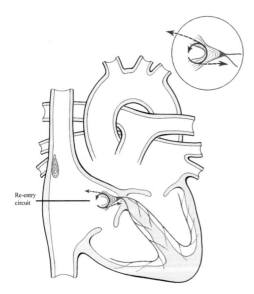

Re-entry circuit

ATRIO-VENTRICULAR NODAL RE-ENTRY CIRCUIT

In adolescents, the circuit may be localised within the atrio-ventricular node ("junction box") where there is an exaggerated imbalance between two areas of this structure allowing the abnormal circuits to occur.

OTHER RE-ENTRY CIRCUITS

The re-entry circuit may be localised within the atria *(atrial flutter or atrial fibrillation)* and occurs when the atria are abnormal, either stretched as a result of being very large or as a result of previous surgical incision. Ventricular tachycardia may occur as a late consequence of complex congenital heart disease or it may occur in otherwise a structurally normal heart. It may have an underlying genetic cause and run in families and occur at stress or exercise.

The management depends on the type of heart rhythm, how often it occurs and how severe are the symptoms. A recording of the abnormal heart rhythm is very important, particularly if and when it needs to be stopped by some medicines.

The most frequent type of arrhythmias in children whose hearts are normal are the first two. If the episodes are short lasting and infrequent, then no regular medicines are required. Many children learn tricks to alter the conduction in the two parts of the pathway, to slow or stop the fast heart rate. Ones that are frequently successful are slow, but deep breathing; trying to make your ears pop, by taking a deep breath in, pinching your nose, closing lips tightly and trying to blow air out, perhaps with your thumb stuck in your mouth; a cold fizzy drink, drunk quickly; splashing cold water on your face or putting an ice pack (frozen peas wrapped in a damp towel) on your face; making oneself gag by putting a finger on the back of the tongue. These episodes, if long lasting, may produce tiredness, discomfort and chest pain. They can almost always be stopped very reliably by an intravenous injection in the Casualty Department at your local hospital. Again, it is very helpful to get an ECG recording during one of these episodes.

If the episodes are more frequent, or cause the child to feel unwell, then regular medications may be required to reduce the chances of them occurring and also to reduce the speed at which the heart responds. The type of medicine and the length of treatment will vary greatly.

If symptoms are very troublesome or severe (causing episodes of collapse and loss of consciousness), the response to medicines is poor, or patients do not wish to take regular medicines for many years, a special catheter test (an electro-physiological test) may be planned. This is like a catheter test. It is usually undertaken under general anaesthesia in children. Fine electrical catheters are positioned in the various part of the heart, the local electrical signals recorded and the fast heart beat is brought on.

The abnormal electrical connection can be localised and if it is a safe distance from the usual conducting system, then it can be modified using radiofrequency energy

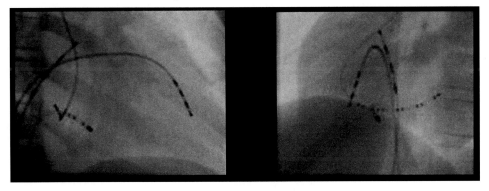

Left: X-ray of electro physiology wires being steered into the heart.

which produces a very localised area of heat damage (called *ablation*).

This procedure lasts for 2 to 4 hours and can be quite complex. There is a small risk of slow heart rate occurring but the results have been really very encouraging. This technique is easy to do in somewhat bigger children after the age of 4 to 5 years.

If it is successful, then medicine can stop and the youngster discharged from follow-up. This has been one of the very exciting developments over the past 5 years in paediatric cardiology.

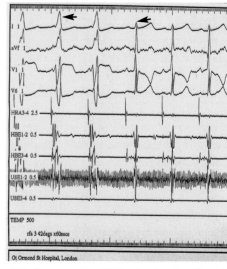

Ablation procedure ECGs showing the effect of the radio frequency pulses on the electrical pathways in the heart (arrowed).

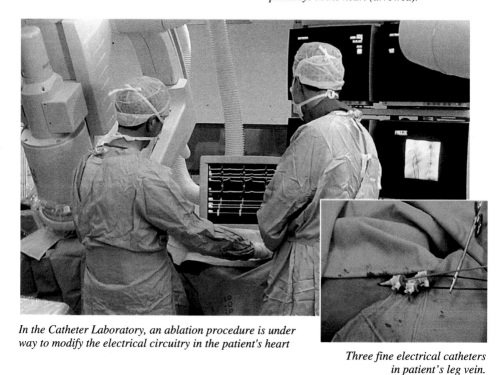

In the Catheter Laboratory, an ablation procedure is under way to modify the electrical circuitry in the patient's heart

Three fine electrical catheters in patient's leg vein.

6 WHEN IT'S TIME FOR AN OPERATION

When the time comes for an operation, it is best to be as well prepared as possible so that you in turn can help your child. You may have already been in the ward. You may have thought how frightening it all looks; all that machinery with flickering lights and alarms going off, with nurses and doctors rushing round all looking very busy, children attached to strange equipment, tubes and wires everywhere and babies hardly visible amongst it all! To the uninitiated this is exactly how it seems!

By this time you will have had a chance to find out what is wrong with your child's heart and what the operation involves.

If you have not been able to do so and your own doctor at home has not been able to help (in such a specialised subject, not every general practitioner may know about all the recent advances in heart surgery) do not hesitate to get in touch with the doctors at the hospital. They will be very happy to explain the situation to you, and will always discuss the forthcoming operation with you in detail.

Your local Parents' Support group will also be able to help you by introducing you to a parent whose child has had heart surgery. See Chapter 17 for where to find more information.

Giving your consent

It is not unusual to have doubts about giving consent for such a big operation to be performed on your child. If he is limited considerably by his heart defect, the decision to give consent will probably be easier than if, to all intents and purposes, your child is leading a normal active life.

However, if the doctors have explained that an operation is necessary, it will usually be because your child's defect, if not corrected before he is much older, will cause considerable damage to his heart muscle or lungs. Unfortunately, there are still some defects which cannot be totally corrected. It may be that the purpose of

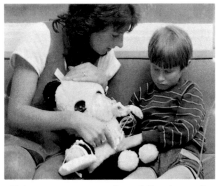

Giving your consent requires a full understanding of the proposed operation. Your child will need to be involved in this if he is old enough to understand what is going to happen.

the operation is to improve, but not to correct. This is termed a 'palliative' procedure. Your doctors will not advise an operation unless they and their colleagues feel that it will help your child to lead an easier and happier life. If your child is older, it is important that he too understands what is planned and agrees.

When the operation is planned, the process of consent is often spread over several weeks or months involving consultations in the outpatients department. However, if the operation is urgent, this process is naturally shortened. It is extremely important for you to ask the doctors to explain simply and carefully to you, the problems and the possible risks and complications that might be involved in the treatment, whether this is for an operation, or for a catheter procedure.

In recent years, there have been enormous advances in cardiac surgery, so that not only can treatment now be undertaken very much more safely than hitherto, but also, conditions previously too complicated to be operable may now be improved. Sadly, occasionally, problems can occur as doctors attempt to improve a child's condition.

To obtain knowledge to deal with these situations and to continue to make advances, it is sometimes helpful for learning if research is undertaken during routine surgery, or catheterisation. You may be approached to ask if you would consent to be involved in such research. It is important that any

procedures proposed are fully explained to you. These will have been carefully reviewed and approved by the hospital's ethical committee process.

It is as a result of this type of research that so much progress has been made and from which so many children now benefit. If you are asked to help, please think carefully and consider how you might be helping other children as well as your own.

Getting used to the hospital. What shall I tell my child?

If your child is old enough to talk, then talk to him about going into hospital. The older he is, the longer he needs to get used to the idea. He will probably have been in hospital before, so remind him of the 'pleasant' things about his stay or what the

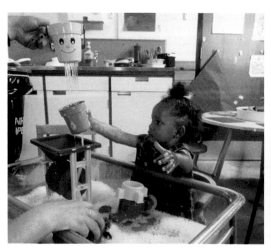

The Playroom is a friendly place where children can relax and get used to being in hospital.

doctors or nurses did. Let him play out these situations with his teddy. Stick a plaster on teddy's leg or chest for example. Buy a toy stethoscope and let him listen to teddy's chest. Playmobile have sets of play people and equipment for hospital work and operating theatre. These are very useful in getting children to play their forthcoming hospital stay.

If he is old enough to understand about his heart being abnormal, then you can tell him that his heart is going to be made better so that he does not get 'puffed out' for instance. Tell him as much about the operation as you think he can understand and answer all his questions honestly. Do not try to change the subject in order to spare his feelings. It is far better for him to talk about his fears than to keep them bottled up. You may say that most children seem to forget all about what happens during this time and that you will be staying in the hospital near him making sure that he is all right.

The Day before the Operation

Your child will be admitted the day before his operation as many of the tests will have been carried out beforehand. It is often quite a busy day so it is useful to have had a look around the unit and the ward beforehand when you have been up at outpatients if that is possible.

The day before admission, let him pack a special bag with some of his favourite toys and make sure to include any 'comforters', blankets, special feeding cups or bottles, etc.

When you arrive you will be shown to the ward, which may not necessarily be the one in which he will be nursed post-operatively. You will be able to meet all the staff and have a chance to ask them any questions that bother you. (see Chapter 8 *Who's Who in Hospital* on page 72). A doctor will examine your child and go through his medical history.

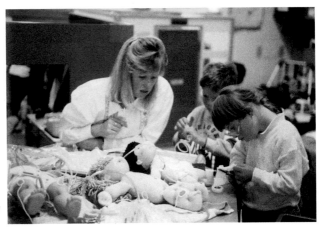

Using play techniques to overcome fears.

The pre-operative tests are important as they will give the doctors information on which to base the post-operative treatment.

They will be:

1. **Blood test** – *blood will be taken from a vein in the arm in order to match up the blood to be used for the operation. If your child is blue this may be difficult, and may have to be repeated as the blood tends to clot very quickly.*

2. **Chest X-ray**

3. **Electrocardiogram** *(ECG)*

4. **Echocardiogram**

5. **Throat swab** – *a sterile cotton wool bud is wiped over the back of the throat and is sent to the laboratory to ensure that there is no infection.*

6. **A urine specimen** *may also be tested to rule out infection. If your child is not 'potty trained', a plastic bag is stuck to the genital area to catch the urine.*

You will meet the surgeon who is part of the team who will be performing the operation. He will explain in detail, with diagrams if necessary, what he plans to do and then will ask you to sign a form saying that you consent to the operation. Sometimes pre-admission clinics are held in the preceding weeks if travelling distance is not too far. If that is the case, you may be admitted on the day of the operation.

You will also, on this day, be shown the Intensive Care Unit (ICU) – see pictures below and overleaf.

This is where your child will return immediately after surgery. You will probably be able to see another child in this room with all the 'machinery' attached. On return from theatre, your child will be attached to a number of pieces of equipment, none of which will cause him much discomfort, although it will be difficult for him to move around.

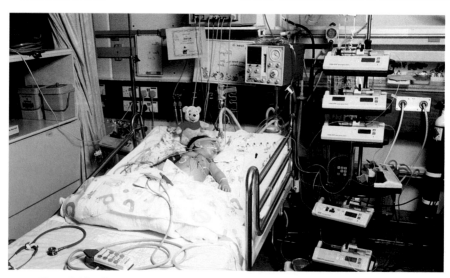

Your child will return to the Intensive Care Unit immediately after the operation.

The Intensive Care Unit (ICU)

Your first visit to the Intensive Care Unit with its array of high technology equipment can be awe-inspiring and it is unlikely that you will be able to take it all in. However, do not be afraid to ask about anything you do not understand.

If your child is old enough and wants to see the Intensive Care Unit, beforehand he may certainly do so, but he should not be forced to see it. Just tell him that he will be in a special room, where there will be doctors and nurses with machines to help him in every way, even to breathe. He will not be able to talk, but he will hear people talking and he will be able to mouth words and the nurses will be able to understand him. Another thing he should know is that for the first day he will not be able to have anything to drink. His mouth will feel very dry, but the nurses will wet his mouth to make it feel better, with a little sponge dipped in water.

Equipment that helps recovery – what it all does – the ICU Room.

If your child is to be 'ventilated', that is, if it is necessary to have his breathing done for him by a machine called a ventilator (and this is quite usual after by-pass surgery and some of the other operations) he will have a tube down his nose or mouth into his windpipe. This allows for the passage of air and oxygen from the ventilator to and from the lungs. To prevent it being dislodged, the ventilator tube may be attached with a band of strapping to your child's forehead.

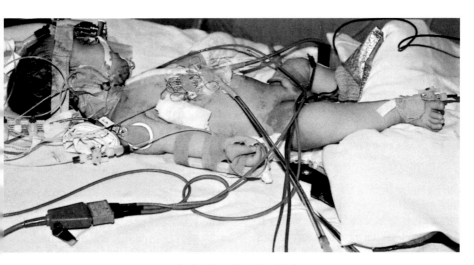

In the Intensive Care Unit

This tube is attached to a longer length of tubing which in turn is connected to the ventilator itself – a small machine standing beside the bed. If your child is able to breathe completely unaided, he will be nursed with an oxygen facemask – or a 'head-box' if he is small enough. Moisture is added to the oxygen, which makes it misty in order to keep chest secretions loose and easier to cough up.

He will have another tube down his nose into his stomach allowing secretions to drain out and so prevent him from being sick. He may have a 'drip' going into a vein on one side of his neck. This is so that he can be fed intravenously for at least the first 24 hours. Both arms may be splinted so that he cannot move them.

There will be further tubes into veins and an artery to provide a means of transfusing him with blood or other fluid, to measure his blood pressure and to give some drugs if necessary. The arterial tube is there for two purposes.

a) Arterial (red) blood can be easily obtained from this tube for sampling purposes. Frequent checks have to be made on the gas and chemical content of the blood to make sure that all the body systems are functioning correctly. This saves your child having frequent needle pricks.

b) The blood pressure can be measured constantly. This takes away the need for your child to be disturbed through frequently having a blood pressure cuff put round his arm or leg. The pressures, along with lots of other vital technical information, are constantly measured through all the various wires attached to your child, and are continuously shown on a television monitor screen.

The operation scar will be either down the middle of the chest or under the arm. On return to the ward there will be a dressing over the wound. Sometimes, young babies may have their sternal wounds left open. Because the heart has been handled for several hours, it will be a bit swollen and may not fit easily enough into the chest cavity for the sternum (breast bone) to be closed. If this is necessary, there will still be a dressing over it and the wound will be stitched up after a day or so. There will be one or two tubes coming out of his chest to drain off any fluid left in the chest cavity or around the heart. The amount is measured and a similar quantity of blood or other fluid is replaced. In those children who have had bypass surgery, there are two 'pacing wires' coming out of the chest which are usually rolled up and attached to the chest in little packets and not used. They are put in routinely at the end of the operation in case the natural pacing mechanism of the heart is temporarily affected by the surgery. The heart may need artificial pacing from a battery driven pacemaker which hangs in a small box at the end of the bed and to which the wires can easily be attached. Finally, post bypass patients have a tube which drains the bladder of all the urine.

The ECMO machine

Very rarely, a child in severe cardio-respiratory failure, may be attached to a special machine called an ECMO *(Extra-Corporeal Membrane Oxygenation)*, which, like the heart-lung bypass machine used in open heart surgery, does the work of the child's heart and lungs. Two *cannulae* (tubes) are inserted in the vein and artery in the neck or left in the chest after surgery. Blood will be drained from the venous side of the heart into the machine, passed through an artificial membrane lung where it is oxygenated and then pumped back into the aorta(the main body artery). This procedure may be continued for several days until the heart and lungs recover. This technique may also be used for babies with various respiratory conditions such as primary pulmonary hypertension of the newborn, meconium aspiration syndrome, bronchiolitis and congenital diaphragmatic hernia. It may also be useful for older children with severe pneumonia, trauma or septic shock as well as after cardiac surgery.

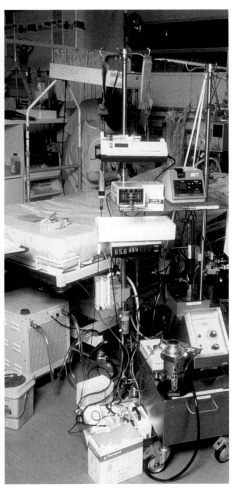

The ECMO machine does the work of the child's heart and lungs.

Ventricular assist devices

These involve inserting a small pump in either or both ventricles and attaching it to a compressor which acts as the power source. They are often referred to as L-VAD. R-VAD, Bi-VAD (left, right or bi-ventricular assist device) As the name suggests they help the ventricle to pump blood around the body.

Aortic balloon pump

This is a tube with an inflatable balloon which is inserted via the femoral artery in the groin up into the aorta and is attached to a machine which helps the heart to provide an adequate circulation.

All these devices are only used when conventional treatment has failed and obviously carry certain risks. If they are necessary, the doctors and nursing staff will give you all the relevant information.

Nitric oxide

This is a gas which, if added to the inspired air, may help to dilate the arteries in the lung and help gas exchange. Some babies with immature lungs or those whose heart defect has meant too much blood going to the lungs may improve if a small amount of nitric oxide is added to the gas going through the ventilator.

Another machine you may see in the Intensive Care Unit is the portable X-ray machine with which chest X-rays are taken while the children are lying flat on their backs.

The hours before the operation

The evening before the operation your child will have a special 'bubble bath' with antiseptic solution in the water to make sure that his skin is really clean. Before he is ready for bed, he may be given a sedative to ensure that he has a good night's sleep. Some hours before the operation, feeds or drinks will be stopped. About one hour before, he will be given his premedication, probably in the form of liquid medicine or a tablet, which will make him sleepy. You will usually be able to accompany your child into the anaesthetic room with one of the ward nurses (NB. Some hospitals may have different arrangements at this time). Tell him that you will see him as soon as the operation is over and try to manage a

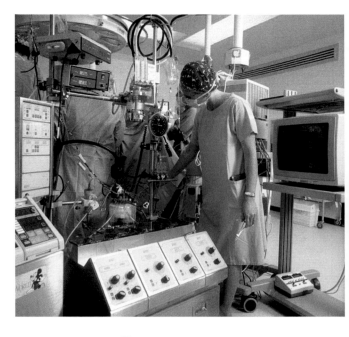

Here is what the Heart-Lung By-pass machine looks like.

This amazing apparatus makes open heart surgery possible and is used in many operations.

big, brave, confident smile, even though you will be probably feeling very frightened and in a state of emotional turmoil inside.

The operation has arrived

For you, now, the next few hours will probably seem the longest hours of your life. If the weather is fine, it is a good idea for you to go out for a walk, or to go shopping, or to visit a museum. Anything, in fact, to occupy your mind and while away the time. You will be given an approximate time to return to the ICU. A bypass operation can take anything from 3-6 hours and the other operations take about 2-4 hours, but delays are frequent – so do not be over anxious. A delay does not mean that anything has gone wrong. The staff know how you are feeling and will try and give you information from time to time. Many hospitals lend their families one of those mobile 'bleeps' so they are able to keep in touch and allay anxiety during this time.

After the operation

When your child is ready to return, a bed which has been specially prepared, is taken to the theatre and he is transferred straight onto it from the theatre operating table. The bed is then wheeled back to the ward. In the ICU, he is attached to all the measuring equipment mentioned earlier. He will then have his chest X-rayed. After all this, which takes about twenty minutes you can see him. He will probably be asleep, because most children are kept well sedated for the first 24 hours. Do not be upset though, if he is awake, because if you ask him later on, you will find that he will remember very little about this first day.

During this period, there will be a nurse and a doctor looking after your child all the time. You will be able to come and visit whenever you like but nobody will expect you to stay for long periods. Your child will be well sedated and probably will remember very little of this experience in ICU. Most ICU units will ask you to check with a member of staff before entering as these are very busy times, with doctors and nurses often having to concentrate specially hard on your child's care. The nurse will be constantly attending your child checking on everything at least every fifteen minutes. Although the machines help the nurses and doctors a great deal, they cannot do the actual nursing!

You will quickly notice that the machines in the ICU keep up a chorus of bleeping noises and that from time to time, alarms appear to go off, adding to your 'stress'. It is easy to be frightened by all this – or to misinterpret the information on the monitors if you are not medically trained. If in doubt, ask someone. The staff will be happy to explain, but try to help them by choosing a moment when they are less busy!

You will notice on occasions that the nurse will encourage your child to cough by applying suction to the tube in the windpipe, the nostrils and the mouth. This is done to prevent pooling of secretions in the lungs and to minimise the onset of chest infection. Chest physiotherapy will be given regularly by the physiotherapist.

ICU nursing goes on throughout the night. You are advised to take advantage of the beds provided for you nearby, because the day will have been mentally very exhausting for you. If, for any reason, the doctors are worried, or there is anything they think you should know, they will contact you. Conversely, if you wake up during the night and want to know how your child is, all you have to do is dial the internal number of the ward and you may talk to the sister or staff nurse in charge.

The next morning after various tests, including blood tests, X-ray and often echocardiograms, tubes in the chest and perhaps the pacing wires will probably be removed. He will be weaned off the ventilator if that has been necessary and once he is breathing on his own then the tube will be removed from his windpipe. He will start having small drinks and later, a light diet.

The rate of progress varies from child to child depending on the severity of the heart defect and the sort of operation performed.

The removal of all the tubes may take up to a week or even longer, so do not be disappointed if your child seems to be taking longer than others. When he does start to drink, the amount of fluid given has to be limited for at least the first 48 hours because if he has too much, the kidneys may not be able to function properly. Therefore, you will be asked to measure all the fluid your child drinks.

Once most of the tubes have been removed your child will be transferred from the Intensive Care Unit to another room. On the third day after the operation he may well be able to sit out of bed or even walk a little.

Gradually, he will return to normal activity, but you will notice that he will be tired and probably rather irritable and miserable. This is a normal reaction – commonly known as 'post-op blues'.

Try to encourage your child to rest as much as possible and he will gradually revert to his normal self.

A few days later, his pacing wires will be removed (if not removed before) and the couple of drain stitches removed. If everything has gone according to plan, your child will probably be allowed home 4-10 days after the operation but it is not uncommon for some to have to stay several weeks. It is very difficult to guarantee the actual date of discharge, so it is better to just wait and see!

During the course of recovery your child will have been given several medicines and it is likely that he will have to take some when he does go home (see Chapter, 13 page 96).

You will be provided with a supply to take with you. You should continue these until your child comes back for his out-patient appointment check-up which will normally be about four weeks after discharge.

IF YOU RUN OUT BEFORE THEN, YOUR OWN DOCTOR AT HOME WILL BE ABLE TO PRESCRIBE MORE. PLEASE DO NOT FORGET!

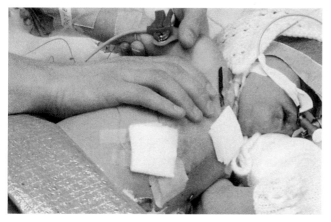

Physiotherapy is an important part of recovery after a heart operation.

Possible Complications

As with all procedures, there may be some complications. Some of the more common ones are as follows:

(a) After Surgery

1. BLEEDING

Immediately after the operation, especially if it is not the child's first operation, there is the possibility that he will bleed excessively from his operation site. The drains in the wound have to be kept clear so that the blood may drain freely and more often than not the bleeding will stop spontaneously. If however it persists, it may be necessary for the child to return to the operating theatre for the surgeon to investigate and maybe put extra stitches into the heart or blood vessels. There's always enough blood ready to give the child to replace what he has lost and it is not usually a major problem.

2. ARRHYTHMIAS

Sometimes during cardiac surgery the natural pacing mechanisms in the heart become swollen, resulting in an irregular or slow heart beat. Temporary 'pacing' with the use of an external pacemaker may be necessary and in rare instances a permanent pacemaker may be required *(Also see Chapter 5, page 45).*

Occasionally the heart beats very fast and medicines are given on a regular basis to slow it down. Another treatment may involve cooling the child to slightly below normal temperature so that the heart has less work to do.

3. PARALYSED DIAPHRAGM

Sometimes during complex surgery in the chest, the phrenic nerve may be damaged or become swollen. This has an effect on the movement of the right or left diaphragm, which in turn affects the breathing pattern of the child. In children under one year of age this may cause difficulties in weaning them from the ventilator and often it may be necessary to 'plicate', that is to fix the diaphragm, to stop its abnormal movement. This necessitates another small operation.

4. INFECTION

Infection is always a danger after any operation. Because after cardiac surgery the child is ventilated by an artificial airway, chest infections can be a problem. These can be treated with appropriate antibiotics. Should the infection get into the bloodstream (septicaemia) then a longer course of antibiotics might be required. Very rarely the wound may become infected. Again antibiotics will be given, but if the infection is deep within the wound it might be necessary for the child to return to the operating theatre and have the whole wound area cleaned and restitched.

5. RENAL FAILURE

After a long operation carried out with the heart lung bypass machine the kidneys may not be able to excrete fluid and waste matter as well as they should.

Following surgery the amount of urine passed each hour is carefully measured. If the amount passed is not sufficient then peritoneal dialysis might be introduced. This involves inserting a fine tube into the

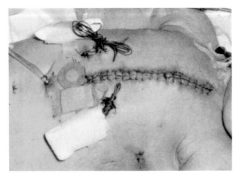

Peritoneal dialysis catheter in the upper abdomen. Coiled pacing wire are also shown.

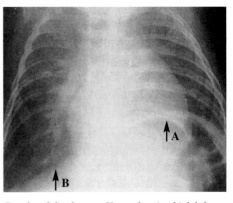

Paralysed diaphragm: X-ray showing high left diaphragm "A" and normal right diaphragm "B".

abdomen and washing out the peritoneal cavity with fluid, which draws out the impurities in the blood. A measured amount of fluid is inserted and then drained out each hour until the kidneys start working properly.

6. CHYLOTHORAX

The fine vessels that carry lymph fluid from the abdomen into the big vein at the top of the chest may be bruised as a result of operations, or may be over stretched and distended as a result of high pressure within the vein into which they feed. These fine vessels are thin walled and carry fluid, particularly fat absorbed from the intestine into the circulation. The largest is called the *thoracic duct*. If a leak occurs, it occurs into the space *(pleura)* between the chest wall and the lung. It may need draining with a tube and an alteration in the diet to change the type of fat given to one that is absorbed more directly into the blood stream rather than using these lymphatic vessels. It is more likely to occur in small babies with

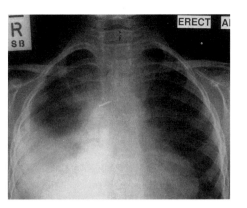

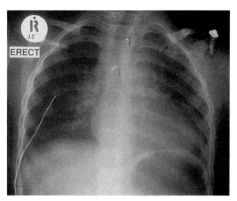

Chylothorax 1 - the white area on the left of the picture indicates fluid which causes this condition.

Chylothorax 2- the white line on the left side of the picture is the drain tube and the fluid is reduced.

complex problems. The special diet is often needed for up to four weeks. Sometimes, the bowel has to be rested completely and intravenous feeding is then used. Occasionally, the damaged vessels need to be tied off by an additional operation.

7. VOCAL CORD PARALYSIS

The nerve supply to the vocal cord runs from the neck down into the chest around the duct between aorta and the lung artery before returning into the neck and the throat. It can become bruised and damaged by complex operations in the area of the large arteries. This can cause the voice to be weak and produce noisy and difficult breathing. In time it usually improves.

8. BRAIN DAMAGE

This is the complication about which everyone worries the most, but fortunately it is rare. If the child is unstable post-operatively with very low blood pressure

then there is a possibility that the brain may not be receiving an adequate blood supply, despite all the appropriate treatment. This may cause unconsciousness or convulsions. This is usually short lived and most children make a full recovery. Another reason for convulsions may be abnormal blood chemistry, such as low blood sugar or calcium levels. Blood is checked regularly for these and other levels and the situation corrected as necessary.

High temperatures may cause convulsions, especially in the young child. For that reason you will notice that if the child's temperature is increasing, then every effort is made to cool him down. If the child has suffered from any of these complications, a check electroencephalogram – a test on brain waves – and often a brain scan are performed to see if any damage to the brain can be detected. In the instance where there is evidence of damage, usually it is of short duration with good recovery. Sadly in very rare instances, there may be lasting problems.

(b) After Cardiac Catheterisation

1. ARTERIAL BLOCKAGE

Occasionally, arteries go into spasm after catheters have been inserted and a clot develops there, reducing the blood flow to the limb. Thinning medicine in the form of Heparin, Streptokinase or TPA is used to disperse this clot. Very occasionally, the artery would need to be explored with surgery and the clot removed with a special balloon catheter.

2. EMBOLUS

Very occasionally, small clots can develop on the tip of the catheter, fly off into the circulation and cause blockage of a small blood vessel. The areas of concern are the blood vessels that go to the brain and very occasionally, a stroke may occur. This is more likely in complex catheter procedures in sick children, whose blood may be very thick as a result of their being very blue.

3. BRUISING

After the catheter is removed, the bleeding usually stops, but it may sometimes restart. This will cause blood loss, and swelling under the skin which can be quite painful. With pressure, this will settle, but the stiffness in the leg will take a week or so to settle and the bruising, a few weeks to improve. Delay in undertaking sporting activities is usually advised.

4. DEVICE EMBOLISATION

Coils or plugs are chosen to block the abnormal vessels, or holes. Occasionally they may move, either during the procedure, or over the following night. If the former, they can be retrieved using a special 'lasso' type catheter, and then a different type of coil plug is used to block the vessel. If it occurs later, then the child will need to return to the catheter laboratory for this procedure to be undertaken.

Occasionally, devices cannot be removed and can be left in safely, blocking small vessels in the lungs. At other times, an operation may be necessary to close the abnormal vessel or hole, and remove the device at the same time.

5. OVER STRETCHING OF VESSELS

A narrow artery can be stretched by a balloon catheter and it may in addition be held open with a metal coil called a stent. Occasionally, blood vessel walls will leak when this is being performed and very occasionally, an urgent operation is necessary to repair the leaking blood vessel.

NB. IMPORTANT NOTE TO PARENTS:

Please note that by telling you about these complications we do NOT mean they will happen, merely that they *might* be a possibility. Please discuss any anxieties you have with the team looking after your child.

7 FUNDAMENTAL FACTS
for Parents about Children's Heart Problems

HEART FAILURE

This is the term used when the pumping action of the heart is insufficient to meet the needs of the body. It means that the heart muscle has extra work to do and help is often needed with medicines and sometimes operations.

It is one of the common presentations of heart problems in children. It is important to reassure everyone that it does not mean that the heart is going to stop or that a serious collapse is likely to occur. However there are different degrees of heart failure ranging from mild to severe.

There are many causes of this extra work and they can occur on their own or in combination with each other. Common examples are large holes between the two sides of the heart, significantly narrow or leaking valves, or weak heart muscle. As a result extra fluid and salts are retained in the body making the lungs wetter, heavier and stiffer than normal and causing breathlessness.

In small babies and children feeding is frequently difficult with slow weight gain and frequent chest infections.

In the older child, tiredness and increasing breathlessness on exercise occur. Sometimes the extra fluid produces abdominal discomfort and swelling and occasionally a puffy face.

TREATMENT – These children can be greatly helped by medicines and depending on the cause may need an operation.

ENDOCARDITIS

This is a serious infection ('ITIS') of the endocardium, which is the smooth lining of the heart. It is extremely rare in normal hearts, and is even uncommon in those that are abnormal. In conditions where there is an abnormal blood flow in the heart, turbulence occurs. This causes some localised thickening and roughening of the lining layer.

If bacteria get into the blood stream in large quantities, they may land in the crevices of this rough area and cause an

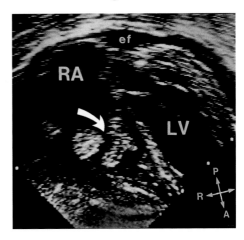

Echocardiogram showing 'vegetation' caused by endocarditis (arrowed).

infection which may be seen as a 'vegetation' on an echocardiogram scan – see picture. This produces general effects such as tiredness, lethargy, fever, weight loss and sweating, and local effects by damage to the area of the infection, particularly relating to the heart valves. In addition, small clots of blood, which may form on the infected areas, can fly off into the circulation and produce problems.

Endocarditis is extremely rare in pulmonary stenosis and atrial septal defects, but is relatively more common in aortic stenosis, mitral valve problems, ventricular septal defects and persistent arterial duct.

Management involves confirming the diagnosis, by taking repeated blood tests to look for the bacteria, echocardiography to look for 'vegetation' followed by large doses of powerful antibiotics, usually into one of the veins for a long period of time (between two to six weeks). Shorter courses are frequently followed by several weeks of oral antibiotics. During much of this time the child will need to be in hospital. The majority of children make a slow recovery.

However, occasionally the infection does not clear and the possibility of urgent surgery may need to be considered.

This is a serious illness and any procedures which are known to be associated with bacteria getting in the blood stream should be covered by giving the patient a large dose of antibiotics beforehand. Most units have cards which they give to parents to show to local doctors and dentists.

Fashions like body piercing and tattooing, should also be avoided.

ACQUIRED HEART DISEASE

Occasionally hearts that have been normal are damaged by acute illness:-

Kawasaki's disease – this produces a generalised inflammation of blood vessels with a high fever lasting longer than 5 days, sore mouth, enlarged lymph glands, inflamed eyes, red rash which eventually peels and a very miserable child. The blood vessels that supply the heart muscle, may be enlarged producing dilatation or aneurysms. The majority settle completely. In others, the vessels remain large and long term treatment with blood thinning medicines e.g. Aspirin is necessary.

The complications can be reduced by giving a special protein (immunoglobulin) early in the illness. It is likely that the usual advice given to adults with regard to smoking, weight, fat intake and lifestyle will be stressed in the long term care of adults who had this illness as children.

The cause is unknown but it is likely to be an abnormal response to a common infection.

Rheumatic fever – this is the commonest acquired heart disease world wide and is an abnormal response to a sore throat with a streptococcus. The infection produces inflammation of heart valves, heart muscle and the joints. Recurrent episodes are likely and each one increases the chance of significant valvar damage. Regular antibiotic treatment with Penicillin is given until young adulthood to reduce the chance of further infections.

Viral myocarditis – the heart muscle can occasionally become weak as a result of a general viral infection. It is likely that most cases resolve spontaneously without becoming a clinical problem. Occasionally, severe damage occurs which requires drugs to support the heart muscle and perhaps to damp down the effect of the viral illness. Very rarely, the illness is so severe that recovery is not possible and heart transplantation may be considered.

'OPEN HEART' SURGERY

This term is used to describe operations on the heart and major blood vessels when the heart's action needs to be stopped. During the operation, the blood supply to the body is able to be continued by an artificial pump and oxygenator known as a heart/lung bypass (page 58), which temporarily takes over the job of both organs. This is connected to the veins and arteries by a set of tubes and maintains the blood supply to the body while the operation on the heart is being undertaken. The temperature of the child's body is frequently cooled (called *hypothermia*) to reduce the demands of the body and a special salt solution *(cardioplegia)* is used to protect the heart muscle.

The children are anaesthetised, have several fine tubes inserted into the large veins, often in the neck, to be able to measure pressures within the veins and to give drugs. A line is placed in an artery, usually in the arm or sometimes the leg to measure the blood pressure. The operations are usually carried out through the breast bone (sternum) and take between three and five hours depending on the complexity. The heart/lung machine and its tubes are connected to the patient, maintaining the blood supply to the body and the heart is relaxed. The heart chamber or vessel is then opened, the defect repaired and following this, the walls are sewn up. The heart is then stimulated and takes over the circulation and gradually the bypass machine can be withdrawn.

Additional tubes (drains) are left around the heart to ensure that any excess fluid is removed, and frequently fine pacing wires are sewn on to the front surface of the heart. Through these an electric current can be given to increase the patient's heart rate if it is a bit slow.

On return to the ward, most children will still require help with their breathing with the aid of a ventilator described earlier and will have the small tubes coming out of their chest to allow the fluid to drain away.

Over the next hours and days these will gradually be removed and the child will leave the Intensive Care Unit. Many children will need to take several medications following their discharge from hospital. This is routine practice. Frequently over the subsequent weeks and months these will be able to be reduced following review in out-patients.

CLOSED SURGERY

This describes operations where the heart's action does not have to be stopped. These are often undertaken through the side of the chest. Repair of coarctation, ligation of the arterial duct, banding of the lung artery to reduce excessive blood flow, stretching of pulmonary and aortic valves and shunt procedures to increase the blood flow into the lungs are all examples of closed surgery.

The child is anaesthetised, frequently there are drips in the side of the neck or the arm; a small tube is often put in an artery to measure the pressure. The incision is usually under the arm running along the line of the ribs. The underlying lung is moved to one side and the defect repaired or a shunt created. The lung is allowed to move back. A small tube is inserted into the chest to allow air and fluid to drain out and to ensure that the lung expands fully. On return to the ward the children may be ventilated, particularly if they are young.

Occasionally closed surgery is under-taken through the breast bone when the blood flow coming into the heart can be reduced allowing straight forward procedures to be undertaken. This is called 'inflow occlusion'.

VALVE REPLACEMENT

If a valve is very abnormal, repair may not be possible and it may need to be replaced. There are many types of new valves which are selected according to the different jobs that have to be done in the heart. However, artificial valves do not grow with the child and may need replacing as growth occurs over the years. The largest possible valve is therefore inserted at the first operation. All these operations require open heart surgery.

In the mitral position, it is usual to use an artificial metal and plastic valve, for example a *Carbomedics valve*. The disadvantage with artificial valves is that the blood needs to be thinned with anti-coagulants to prevent small clots forming on the metal and plastic parts. These clots may then fly off into the circulation, or cause the valve itself to stick, or leak. The degree of blood thinning required, needs to be checked by regular tests. 'Finger-prick' home testing machines are being introduced to make this task easier to manage.

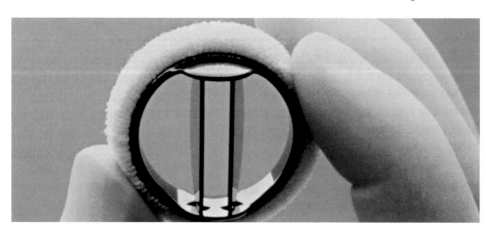

A Carbomedics artificial heart valve.

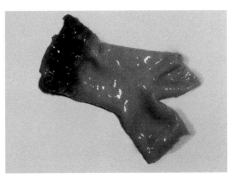 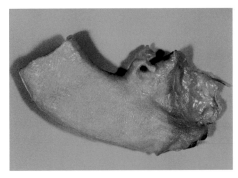

A homograft is a human donated valve. Left is a pulmonary homograft. An aortic/homograft is shown right. Photos: courtesy of Royal Brompton Hospital.

The aortic valve can be replaced by a similar type of artificial valve. Substituting the abnormal aortic valve with the patient's own pulmonary valve and putting an artificial donor valve *(known as a 'homograft')* into the low pressure pulmonary position is another possibility. This uses the patient's own native valve tissue in the high pressure, high stress side of the circulation and has given very encouraging results in the medium term (the **Ross Procedure**). These latter operations avoid the use of anticoagulants which is particularly beneficial in children and young women.

The tricuspid valve may require replacement with a plastic and metal valve, but occasionally a *homograft* may be used here (see above).

In contrast, a pulmonary valve that is very abnormal, may be removed completely, as the right-sided pump chamber copes very well with the degree of extra work that the backflow of blood from the lung produces.

Sometimes this leak is excessive and a new pulmonary valve would need to be inserted. This usually is a *homograft* which can be sewn on to the top of the right ventricle.

A valve replacement is a more major undertaking in children than in adults. It requires enough space within the heart to insert the valve. Regular long term follow-up is required **and antibiotic prophylaxis is extremely important.**

CONDUITS

A conduit is an artificial tube that carries blood, usually with a valve within it. The use of conduits has made previously inoperable heart disease treatable. The valve may be a *homograft* (a human valve) or a *xenograft* (pig or calf valve). Conduits are used to insert a valve which was completely missing, or when it is impossible to repair the patient's own one, or to bypass a severe narrowing that cannot be relieved directly.

The valve and conduit will not grow. This means that if they have to be inserted in small children they may need to be replaced as the years go by.

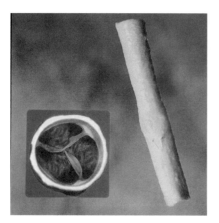
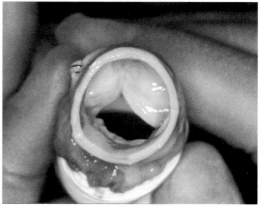

A conduit – an artificial tube and valve which is used where the patient's own valve is completely missing, or needs to be replaced. The two shown are xenografts which originate from a pig or a calf.

Conduit operations are often postponed until the child is between four and eight years when a larger size can be used. However, even then many of these will require a further operation, because of the development of narrowing over many years.

Long term follow-up is required, as is antibiotic prophylaxis.

TRANSPLANTATION
Heart, Heart and Lung, Lung

The first paediatric heart transplantation was performed in 1967 but due to problems with rejection, interest declined until new drugs to control rejection became available in the late 1970s. Since then, heart, heart and lung, and lung transplantation have become a well established treatment for children with end-stage heart and/or lung disease.

If the problem is only the heart, but the lungs are good, then only the heart is transplanted. If the lungs are badly damaged, or because of abnormal blood vessels (high blood pressure in the lungs or severe narrowing), either both lungs are transplanted – or heart and lungs together.

Transplantations are only carried out in a few centres and therefore the children and families will need to be assessed by the transplant team. This means meeting the teams of doctors, nurses, and social workers who are involved in the operation and the care afterwards.

During the assessment time, additional investigations will be undertaken and the families will have the opportunity to meet others who have had transplants. This enables them to learn about the benefits of transplantation, but also to hear about the difficulties, problems and implications of having this sort of treatment. They can then finally decide if this would be right for their child.

The waiting time for the actual transplant is very variable as the supply of new hearts and particularly lungs is unpredictable. In addition the team have to match up not only size but blood group. This waiting often causes a great strain on all members of the family.

When a suitable organ is available the family are informed and have to return to the transplant unit as quickly as possible. Good planning is necessary for this to take place. The operation lasts from four to six hours, sometimes even longer and frequently happens at night. After the operation, the child usually returns to a special ward in order to reduce the risk of infection.

The main problems after transplantation are suppressing the body's attempts to reject the new organs and preventing infection. To do this powerful drugs are used and in the first days after the operation these are given in very high doses. During this time, access is restricted to prevent the introduction of infection. As soon as possible all tubes and lines are removed and the child is mobilised. Over the next weeks the optimum doses of the anti-rejection drugs are worked out. The child usually recovers quickly and the majority can be discharged after two to four weeks, but frequent out-patient visits are required in the next few weeks, after which the need for follow-up is gradually reduced.

Rejection of the new organ occurs in almost all patients at some stage or another, most frequently within the first few months. Rejection is assessed by temperature changes, breathing tests, ECGs and echocardiograms and in some cases by taking small pieces of heart muscle or lung tissue and looking at them under microscopy (biopsies). To prevent rejection, anti-rejection medicine needs to be given life long, but the doses can usually be gradually reduced as long as the progress is satisfactory.

The long term results from transplantation are improving, but remain better for isolated heart transplant than for transplants involving the lungs. This is because the lungs are more immunologically active organs and therefore more prone not only to rejection but also to infection. Side effects of the powerful drugs used may in some cases be a problem, e.g. high blood pressure, kidney problems or excess hair, but are generally well tolerated. Medicines will need to be altered over the years and blood tests performed regularly to check that the right doses are being given.

Despite the optimal use of anti-rejection medicines, chronic low grade rejection remains a significant problem. In the long term, this will eventually damage the new organs, gradually reducing their functions. This means transplantation is not a cure, rather a palliative procedure, and therefore a major step. The family and child need to be aware of the difficulties associated with such a major operation both in the short and long term. It can, however, mean a significantly improved quality of life for the children with very severe problems for a number of years. Hopefully, the long-term results will continue to improve as new drugs and clinical techniques become available.

WHO'S WHO IN HOSPITAL
Parent's guide to who does what!

CHAPTER

8

1. PEDIATRIC CARDIOLOGIST – is the doctor who will find out exactly what is wrong with your child's heart. He will be in charge of your child's care while he is in hospital and also in outpatients. He will arrange the cardiac catheterisation and echocardiogram.

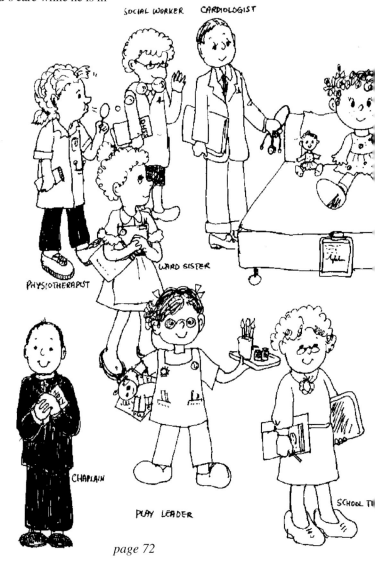

SOCIAL WORKER   CARDIOLOGIST

PHYSIOTHERAPIST

WARD SISTER

CHAPLAIN

PLAY LEADER

SCHOOL T...

2. PEDIATRIC CARDIAC SURGEON
– (sometimes known as 'Mr' rather than 'Dr'). This is the doctor who will perform the operation on your child's heart and who will talk to you before and after the operation to explain what has to be done. Each of these doctors has a team to help him. They are Registrars and House Officers who will all be involved in the care of your child, performing the investigations, and helping with the operations.

3. INTENSIVIST
– a specialist doctor who will look after your child while he is in the intensive care unit immediately after the operation.

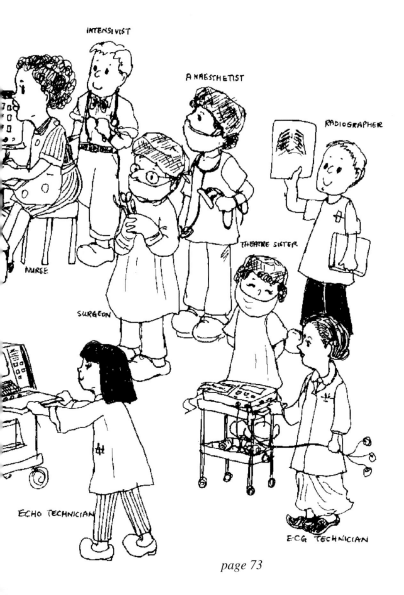

INTENSIVIST

ANAESTHETIST

RADIOGRAPHER

NURSE

THEATRE SISTER

SURGEON

ECHO TECHNICIAN

ECG TECHNICIAN

4. ANAESTHETIST – this is a doctor who administers the anaesthetic to your child so he is asleep and free of pain during and immediately following operations and catheter procedures.

This doctor may also look after the ventilation of your child if at any stage help needs to be given with his breathing.

5. THEATRE SISTER OR STAFF NURSES – these nurses assist the surgeons while they operate on your child.

6. PERFUSIONIST – a technician who looks after the heart/lung bypass.

7. ECG TECHNICIAN – makes an electrocardiographic recording of your child's heartbeat and will be involved in the follow-up and checking of pacemakers.

8. ECHO TECHNICIAN – this is the person who performs the ultrasound sound wave scans.

9. CATHETER LAB TECHNICIAN – this is the person who records the pressures and maintains the equipment for the cardiac catheterisation procedures.

10. WARD SISTER or CHARGE NURSE (if male) – is responsible for the ward and the nurses working in it.

11. STAFF NURSE – a trained nurse who will look after your child while he is in hospital.

12. STUDENT NURSE – is there to learn and to gain experience and is supervised by the staff nurses and sisters.

13. PLAY LEADER – is there to help entertain your child and through play help him to understand what the doctors and nurses are doing and helps to prepare your child for the operation.

14. WARD RECEPTIONIST – this is the person who often answers the telephone, helps the doctors and nurses with a great deal of the paperwork necessary on the ward.

15. PHYSIOTHERAPIST – will encourage your child to expand his lungs and breathe properly after his operation and will also help him to get out of bed and move normally.

16. RADIOGRAPHER – takes X-ray pictures of your child's chest either in the X-ray department or with a portable machine in the ward.

17. LABORATORY TECHNICIAN – is someone who visits the ward to take blood specimens from your child for special tests.

18. PHARMACIST – makes up all the medicine prescribed for your child by the doctors and is based in the hospital.

19. CHAPLAIN – you will find that there are representatives of all the main religious denominations visiting the hospital. If you wish to see one of them, just ask your ward sister or charge nurse, who will arrange it.

20 SOCIAL WORKER – if you have any problems, social or financial concerning your child or the rest of the family, a social worker will be available to discuss these with you and to offer help from many sources.

9 | REACTIONS & FEELINGS
Your own and of those around you

DISCOVERY

When parents are expecting the birth of a child, there is a great feeling of excitement and elation, new hopes for the future, joy and anticipation. But behind these happy feelings, there is a dark shadow. What if there is something wrong with our baby? Most people put this thought out of their minds, so it is a terrible shock to most of us when we learn our child has a heart condition.

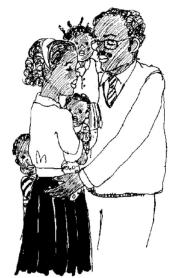

When this happens to us – and our child – it is difficult to accept: 'Why me?' you may ask, a question which we assure you, has no answer yet, although in the future some of the research currently being done may yield some clues.

SORROW

When you discover you have a child with a heart problem it would be unusual not to feel deep unhappiness. The natural way the body copes with this is through tears - a good way to release the pent-up emotions of sorrow and despair. You may try to hold back your tears for fear of embarrassing others – or because you think you may not be able to stop. But don't be. It is not only acceptable but good to share your sorrow, and you will probably feel better for it. A word for fathers, here. Unfortunately the idea of men shedding a tear in our western society has in some way become taboo. You are meant to keep a 'stiff upper lip', come what may. This is a pity because it denies you one of nature's ways of coping with your agony. So take our advice, find a quiet corner and let it all go. You will feel better able to cope after – and you will be more able to support your partner.

ANGER

Anger is another emotion you may need to deal with. It is natural to want to 'lash out' at others when we feel hurt or cornered. If you have a faith, you may feel angry with God for letting it happen to you. Parents are often angry with themselves, because they think they have damaged their child and they feel guilty.

At times you will feel anger with almost everybody else. Most parents deny their feelings of anger – but it is very, very natural.

It is all right to feel angry at this time. Try and talk it out with caring friends.

SHOCK

Initially, when you first discover your child has a problem you may have overwhelming feelings of panic and despair, and then a kind of numbness.

This is your mind's way of protecting you and allowing in only the amount of pain and upset you can handle.

This shock will only allow you to take in as much information as you, personally, can handle. This means that much of the information that is given to you in the first few days and weeks after your child's diagnosis goes 'right over your head' and you find yourself being unable to take everything in.

The medical staff will usually understand this and will try and give you information in comprehensible chunks. A good idea is to keep paper and pen with you and if you don't understand something – or you are afraid of forgetting it, ask the doctor or nurse talking to you to write information down. This is also a useful memory aid if you suddenly think of something and want to remember it for the next time you are speaking to a member of the medical staff. Our memories are not always good when we are in a state of shock!

The parents who have contributed to this book have experienced these same feelings. We can assure you that they are NORMAL HEALTHY RESPONSES.

As the shock fades away you may experience other feelings

– as if you are living in a bad dream

– you may become forgetful, unable to concentrate (especially problematic for parents at work)

– making decisions may be difficult, because you cannot anticipate the future.

DEPRESSION AND ANXIETY

Experiences of parents of heart children indicate that we all go through a see-saw world of elation, as some new good inform- ation arrives, returning to anxiety and depr- ession as things get worse, perhaps as a result of a chance remark from a member of the medical staff – or the effect of some treatment or other. Then there is an improvement – and, up we go again! Waiting for results of tests – the time before an operation – the wait when it is actually happening – all can be very frightening times.

Being on this emotional 'roller-coaster' is likely to cause you desperate fatigue, depression and even despair. But you **can and will** be able to come to terms with it. The key is to keep talking to people who know what you are going through. **You are less alone than you think!**

Talk to the medical staff at your hospital, especially the nurses and Play Leader.

Get in touch with a parents' organisation (see Chapter 17 later in this book).

You will surely find a sympathetic ear to help you through these anxious times.

GUILT

This is a very difficult feeling to come to terms with. In most cases there is no clear reason why your child was born with a heart defect, but it does not stop you searching for one. You may find yourself asking futile questions in an attempt to rationalise it. Was it the medication I took? What about that cold virus I had? And so on. You might find some comfort from the researchers at the very centre of modern heart research. THEY don't yet know how it happens either, although the work plotting the human genome is beginning to reveal new facts.

So learn to recognise the questions that lead to a sense of guilt. If you could have prevented the heart defect you would have done, wouldn't you?

You and your family are NOT TO BLAME.

Later you will quite often find that you have built new caring friendships with people you hardly knew. And our children, who are much more resilient than most of us imagine, often become more self-reliant as a result of these experiences.

However, do remember to maintain communications with the rest of your family at least by phone. Sometimes even

though things look bleak at the hospital, it is wise to go home for a few hours, if practicable. It is amazing how this can put things back in perspective. It's good for parents and the rest of the family.

FATHERS

For you, a father, the way of coping with your child and with the worry of your child's condition will be different from your partner's. Fathers usually need to hold down a job to earn money to keep the home and family together. If you have to take time off, the effect of this can bring its own severe anxieties, especially if you run your own business or have an unsympathetic employer.

It may mean that you don't have time to take your child to clinic, or to spend much time at the hospital, so responsibility may fall mostly on your partner. Splitting your family in this way can be a great strain on a relationship, especially if you have to

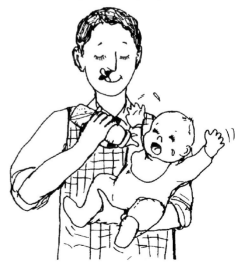

look after your other children as well. You can both help each other by taking time to talk this through together and perhaps occasionally, reversing roles.

Sometimes, fathers find their work acts as a diversion to escape from a distressing situation that is painful to face. This results in having less time for their families than ever before. If you find yourself working too hard, drinking too much, or finding reasons to do things that blot out thinking about your family's problems, or avoid making time for them, recognise the symptoms and talk it through with your partner or a sympathetic friend. Please be assured by the writers that yours is also a key role in the life of your family at this time.

One of the best ways you, as a father, can help is by making a point of visiting your child in hospital as often as you can. Visiting time for parents is usually totally free and most fathers find that evening visits, when they can stay until the child is asleep, fits in well with their work or business commitments.

It will be helpful all round, if you can time your visit when doctors are doing their ward rounds. There are occasions when they would prefer to discuss your child's condition with both parents present. This means you get information first-hand and are able to get answers to any questions you might have. It also helps you feel that you are not being left out.

To have a child with a heart condition is not an everyday problem – it is a situation that is difficult for one person to cope with on their own. So even if you feel your partner is holding up very well, she will appreciate your presence and moral support. You may be amazed at the strength of your partner in these difficult times. You may ask yourself, 'Is she doing so well because she has no alternative?' Try and look for ways to support her – best of all by being there.

It is important to try and restore normality by getting away from the hospital for an hour or so, perhaps by having a meal together.

The hospital staff can always contact you if they need to.

If your partner assumes that you will not want to play a leading part, you as a father, may feel left out and helpless. You may feel you are not needed, that things seem to go along very well without you. In fact,

YOU are needed by *everyone* at this time,

– especially your child and those concerned with the care of your child.

You may find it harder than your partner does to accept the fact that your child has a heart problem. Sometimes, with a new baby you may feel that you do not want to become too attached to your child in case he or she dies. A heart defect is scary, but it has happened. The best thing you can do is to try to accept it, and do the best you can for your child.

In our culture, it is often more difficult for men to express their fears and worries, but talking about them with others is the way to ease the pressure. You will often find great depth of comradeship and an understanding ear from other fathers on your child's ward. Admitting your feelings and sharing them, is the first step towards finding a solution to the problem.

It is better to ask for help than to pretend you don't need it.

You may find that others, too, are helped with their own difficulties, by your willingness to communicate.

REACTIONS OF OTHERS

It is fair to say that the majority of your friends, acquaintances, neighbours – and colleagues at work will be **totally uncomprehending** of the difficulties of having a 'heart' child. Generally you will find that they fall into two sorts.

The first make wildly simplified remarks like 'oh you needn't worry, heart problems – they're easily fixed these days'. The other group over-react in totally the opposite direction 'However will you cope? – my brother's neighbour's little girl is really bad with that', etc., etc. The latter group are often worse than useless and cross the road when they see you coming to avoid being 'upset' by your 'news'.

And you will meet still more who will alarm you by blurting out astonishingly tactless comments.

Comfort yourself by remembering that you understand the reality of the situation in a way that 99.9% of these people never will. Also that there are many who just can't handle your problem – and sadly, simply don't know what to say to you. They react by avoiding you. It is not you they are rejecting – it is your situation.

On the positive side you will probably find a few key people who will step forward to become a tower of strength to you!

You will learn a lot about people when you have a heart child!

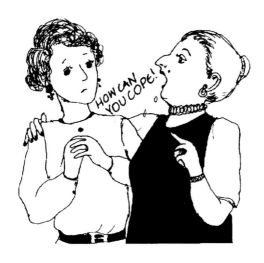

CHAPTER 10
LIVING WITH A HEART CHILD
– Coming home from hospital

Bringing your infant home from hospital is usually a time for celebration. If however, your baby has been diagnosed as having a heart defect, or indeed has already undergone some investigation or surgery, the celebration may be marred with rather more than the usual anxiety. Many parents worry about how they will cope with the full responsibility of caring for their baby. Up until now, this anxiety has been shared with hospital staff, who have always been nearby, if there were questions to be answered.

You may find yourself constantly checking your baby and worrying when, for example, he appears more restless, or seems to be crying more than usual. It is very easy to fall into the trap of attributing every change in your baby's behaviour to his condition, completely forgetting that 'normal' babies also go through periods of fretfulness, lack of appetite, not sleeping and so on. A tip for helping your baby sleep more comfortably is to slightly raise the head of the cot.

Coping alone

The first few months of living with a heart baby are never easy. Even if your baby is a relatively good feeder there is still the problem of coming to terms with his condition to cope with. Before we have a heart baby, the most the majority of us know about the heart is that if it stops, that's it! We are culturally bound to the idea that the heart is the source of life, and therefore the news that there is something wrong with our baby's heart has particularly emotive connotations. Somehow we have to make the leap from knowing very little about how the heart works to understanding that babies with even very complex problems can – and do – survive. And we have to do this at a time when just coping with our baby's needs takes up all our time and energy. If, as in many cases, your baby is a poor feeder, tires easily, falls asleep in the middle of his feed and then wakes up screaming an hour later, and maintains this pattern at night as well, you may well feel as though you are living in a waking nightmare.

The important fact to hold on to during this time is that things *will get better!* As your baby begins to grow you will be able to increase gradually the amount of food he can take and as you get to know him better you will be more relaxed caring for him. Initially, however, it is very hard and if you have an older child, or children, to look after as well, you will need help.

Don't be afraid to ask friends, relatives, your health visitor and of course your partner. If your baby is bottle-fed or you can get him to take milk from a bottle as well, let your man give the evening feed while you have an early night. If friends offer help during day, accept it gladly and ask them to take on some of your household chores as well. If you are feeling in need of a break, leave them with the baby while you go out of the house for a while perhaps with your other child, or go and do some shopping.

Staying Sane!

Babies are remarkable barometers of their mother's emotions, so the more anxious and worried you are feeling the more quickly your baby will 'home in' and react adversely to your feelings, which in turn will obviously affect you. One can very easily get into a seemingly endless cycle of worry and tension; it does help to be aware of this and try and break the cycle before it goes too far. If you feel things starting to get on top of you, try and leave your son or daughter with a trusted friend or relative, even if it is only for an hour and get out. Do anything that makes a change from your normal routine so that you have the opportunity to distance yourself from your problem, even for a short time.

Anxiety is a strong emotion which creates energy: Giving it an outlet, such as a long, brisk walk, gardening, a spell in the gym or, in the absence of anything else, kicking 'hell' out of a cardboard box or similar, (nothing too hard, or it will hurt your feet!). This does help relieve the tension, even if it doesn't do much for the cardboard box!

Parents have found that giving their anxiety an outlet helps them provide a positive, emotionally stable environment for their children. Trying to protect those around you, including your other children and your heart child as he grows older, by keeping your worries to yourself does not usually benefit anyone. Children easily pick up your anxiety and because you do not talk about it they in turn become worried that it is 'too bad' to talk about.

BACK TO NORMALITY

The separation and splitting up of the family while your child is in hospital is one of the things that may cause problems when surgery is hopefully behind you and you come home expecting to be on top of the world and everything to be wonderful. You may not – and it may not be! Many parents talk of returning home and feeling very depressed. If their child has done well they feel guilty about this and cannot understand why they feel so low.

In reality, it is not easy taking back sole responsibility for your child's care, particularly if he may not yet be doing as well as you hoped, when before there was always medical advice and support on tap. Also, for many weeks prior to and during hospitalisation, you will have been living on nervous energy with all other considerations not to do with your child having become irrelevant. It takes quite an adjustment to get back into the routine of work, cooking, shopping etc, which may seem very mundane in comparison.

Coping with a convalescent child who clings to you and is faddy about food, is not easy. Add your other children who may be feeling equally insecure as a result of the separation – and you have a lot to cope with! It is important that you can accept this. Don't ask too much of yourself and your partner – and *do* ask for help and advice if you are worried about anything.

GET HELP!

Let your GP know that you are home from hospital; ask for the Health Visitor to call. There is increasing liaison between Cardiac Units and the local Community Health Visitor so she should know you're home fairly soon anyway but don't wait for her to get in touch.

If you feel concerned that something really is not right with your child, phone the ward of the hospital from where you have been discharged and ask their advice. Staff are aware of how difficult the first few days at home are and will want to help if you are really worried.

Knowing that there is help available to you will help lessen that awful feeling of isolation that many parents feel once they leave hospital and begin the journey home.

When to call the doctor

One of the major worries that parents have during the early months of caring for a heart baby is knowing whether or not he is unwell. As with a normal child one of the best indicators is if he goes off his food. A sudden change in behaviour pattern, e.g. an unusual degree of lethargy or if the baby appears unusually pale or sweaty can also be something to watch. Usually if a baby is taking food normally, there is no cause for concern. Most GP's are very helpful and understand your anxieties, but readily admit that they generally have very few heart children to deal with and so do not always have the information you may be looking for. Many parents find the realisation that their GP is not 'the expert' rather frightening. Who then, can they turn to? It may be helpful to remember that although not a specialist on children's hearts, the GP is still your family doctor, knows a great deal about children's problems, the difference between being 'ill' and 'well' – and does have the responsibility for your child. You should not feel you have to carry the burden alone of deciding when your child is ill. If, for example, you believe your baby is ill, it will help if you can explain to your GP as to why you feel this. If you are requesting a visit at 2 am in the morning (isn't that *always* the time babies and children go from being 'unwell' to 'ill' ?) instead of demanding that a doctor visit, take a deep breath, explain your concern and ask for advice. This puts the onus on the doctor. If your GP does not come out and, having followed advice and instruction, you are still not happy, phone again. If you voice your concern, most doctors will come out, but it is helpful for you if you can describe enough about your child's condition for them to make the choice. Then, the next time when you need to call, you will feel more confident in doing so.

VISITING OUTPATIENTS

Out-patient appointments also allow you to voice any concern you are feeling at your child's condition. Since these may occur only infrequently it is as well to go prepared. If you have several questions to ask, (and who hasn't?) write them down. Many parents complain of suffering a mental block when they are faced with a busy Out-patient Department and a doctor that they may not have seen before. Writing down in advance any questions you want to ask, helps overcome this problem.

Growing up

ACTIVITY, DISCIPLINE

If bringing up a healthy child is difficult enough, raising a child who has a heart condition inevitably presents us with problems we've not even thought of before, let alone had to deal with. We are continually beset with questions: to what extent should I enforce discipline? How much exertion can I allow? What about school, will he cope in a normal school environment?

It sometimes helps to turn the whole situation around and try to change the emphasis. Not 'here is a heart child, what can he do?' but 'here is an ordinary child who happens to have a heart condition, is there anything he cannot do? Young children with heart conditions usually know their own physical limits, more so than adults, and almost never over tax

themselves, therefore it is unnecessary to restrict their activities. Older children with major heart problems may have to avoid over-strenuous exertion and will start to become aware that they cannot always keep up with their playmates at school. Depending on your child's personality, this can cause a great deal of frustration and it may be wise to start thinking of some less physically demanding interest in which to involve him. This should be something at which he can be reasonably good as his ego tends to take a hammering in other areas. For the more physically able child, indoor basketball which uses a smaller area and is played indoors may be an alternative to football or netball when the weather is cold. Drama may serve as a useful outlet for some children. Giving your child a pet of his own to take care of is another possibility. The main thing to strive for, is as full and normal a life as possible and to try and avoid imposing unnecessary restraints. No restrictions need to be put on children with minor defects.

Discipline is basically a matter of teaching a child the rules by which he can live as an acceptable member of society. Therefore, we are doing any child a disservice if we do not teach him these rules. Many parents complain that their 'heart' children are unusually irritable, tearful and lacking in concentration. Clearly, some children do have a lower tolerance level, particularly prior to corrective surgery. Somehow, as parents, we have to try and walk a tightrope between accepting that there are times when our children find just 'carrying on as normal' more than they can cope with – and teaching them that rudeness and temper tantrums are not acceptable modes of behaviour. Tantrums often arise as the result of tiredness and trying to "keep up" with other children. Making times in your daily routine where your child can rest while listening to you read, watching a favourite video or whatever will help establish a pattern of exertion and rest which will help him keep going through the day without it appearing he is being made to rest and therefore being different from his friends.

GOING TO SCHOOL

The first and most common issue you may encounter as your child prepares to start school is, "What will be his needs in coping with the physical environment?"

The second issue that can arise for certain children with heart problems, as it also does for those without them, is what support may be needed for him to fulfill his learning potential. Coping with the physical environment can usually be effectively dealt with by contacting your chosen school before the start of the first term and enlisting the help of the head teacher and class teachers in assessing the best way to overcome any potential difficulties your child may have. These will clearly depend on the severity and nature of your child's heart problem.

Most parents find that schools welcome their children and do try very hard to provide for any extra needs that the child may have, although this is not always the case! If going outside in very cold weather is not advisable, some schools overcome the problem by providing younger children with a job to do indoors, e.g. looking after any classroom pets, watering the plants etc. or it may be possible to choose a friend to keep him company in the classroom or school hall during playtime. Those with severe heart problems may be eligible for a 'classroom assistant', who is available for part of the school day, specifically to help your child. This may in itself cause problems as all children hate being different! The degree of exposure the assistant has will depend on the circumstances. A sensitive helper will blend into the background to avoid being seen to support one child. Obviously an extra pair of hands within any class in this situation is always welcome. You can be sure that if your child is eligible, the school will be more than happy to welcome them and the support they may be entitled to bring with them.

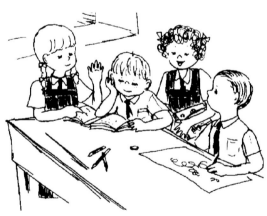

Special Needs and Statementing

As with any group of children, there will be those, including some heart children who have learning difficulties at school. Your Local Education Authority (LEA) has a statutory obligation to assess each child's educational needs and to abide by a clearly set out code of practice in doing so.

This code of practice recommends the general adoption of a staged model of special educational needs. The first 3 stages are based in the school. This means the school has responsibility for making them work, but can, as necessary, call upon the help of external specialists. At stages 4 and 5 the LEA shares responsibility with schools.

The five stages work out approximately as follows:

Stage 1: The class or subject teacher identifies that a child may need some help with his learning and develops an individual learning plan as well as consulting the school's Special Educational Needs (SEN) coordinator.

Stage 2: The school's SEN co-ordinator takes lead responsibility for gathering information and coordinating the child's special educational provision.

Stage 3: Teachers and the SEN coordinator are supported by specialists from outside the school.

Stage 4: The LEA consider the need for a statutory assessment

Stage 5: The LEA consider the need for a statement of special educational needs and, if appropriate, makes a statement and arrange, monitor and review the provision.

A significant proportion of children in any class will be on the SEN register at Stages 1 or 2 at some point in their schooling. Being put onto the register at Stage 1 means that the class teacher is aware that a child is having some difficulties in an area of learning.

Going on to the SEN register acts as a trigger to the class teacher to develop an individual learning plan to assist the child and to raise awareness that there may be a problem which could be temporary or longer term.

For example, children who have to have periods off school due to ill health, will benefit from an individual education plan, because it will help them to catch up with the rest of their class in a structured way.

If after a period of time the child is not making progress, then the decision may be taken to move them to Stage 2, or if it is felt that some outside specialist help is needed, to Stage 3. This whole process of moving the child through the SEN register is done in a very structured way to focus first and foremost on the needs of your child.

HELPING SIBLINGS COPE

It is sometimes difficult for other children in your family to understand why their brother or sister maybe the object of extra attention from grandparents and other relatives or friends. It is natural they may feel some resentment about this and they will find it easier to cope if they are helped to understand why it occurs. This may be particularly the case when your 'heart baby' is first diagnosed. An older brother or sister, if their baby brother or sister's illness is not explained, may feel that they are responsible for the illness because of naturally occurring jealousy at the new arrival. An older child of pre-school age may not understand any more than that the baby is ill but they can be encouraged to help with simple fetching and carrying tasks and be included in bathing and changing rituals. This will help children feel included and less anxious about the strain their parents are clearly under.

When the baby is older, brothers and sisters need to be kept in touch with the situation. If hospitalisation is necessary, they will be better able to cope with the separation from both their parents and sibling if it has been talked over with them, so they know why it has to occur and exactly who will be looking after them while mum and/or dad is away at the hospital.

Outside support

Some people who have never had a sick child, find it very difficult to understand what a strain it can be. It is very difficult to explain the sense of isolation one can feel when faced with the never-ending questions entailed in bringing up a heart baby. Why isn't he putting on weight? What will they say at the next hospital appointment? Is it normal for him to be late sitting up, crawling, walking? Does he seem more breathless, bluer than usual? It seems impossible sometimes to find someone willing to listen to your anxieties for as long as you want to voice them. Friends may expect you to react in a certain way, or they may react in a way you find difficult to accept. You may mention to a friend that you are worried about some aspect of your baby's condition, to have that friend reply that her 'non heart' baby is 'just the same'. If you are looking for a sounding board at that particular time, this quite harmless reply may be reassuring or may be quite incredibly irritating. Other

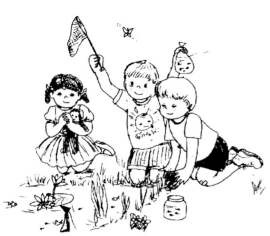

mothers wonder what to say to well-meaning strangers who look at their blue-tinged children and ask if they are wrapped up warmly enough. There will be times when you will feel as if no one understands your problems at all. Do not cut people out of your life because they appear to be out of sympathy with you at a particular time.

The support of others will become more important to you as your child grows, so try not to become so involved in him that you have no room for anyone else. Try to maintain some outside interests. Many parents have found joining a support group helps to put things in perspective. If you are feeling particularly anxious about how your baby will cope as he grows up, seeing another child with an equally severe problem coping well may help ease your fears and encourage you to feel more optimistic about the future.

While your child is small it is almost impossible to picture him as a teenager or adult. Getting him through the first few years seems such a major hurdle, and it can be quite scary looking further into the future – suppose he doesn't have a future? If you are living with this fear, or even if you are feeling very optimistic but still coping with the everyday traumas of living with a heart child, the idea that the day will come when he will no longer need you to speak for him – in an outpatients clinic for example, can be difficult to imagine. But we do owe it to our children to eventually let go of the whole responsibility for their health and well-being and hand it over to them.

One way to begin, is by discussing with your child what he wants to get out of the next outpatient appointment. Is it reassurance, information, what questions does he want to ask? Agree a list and make sure he is the one in charge of it – and that he asks the questions. How soon should you start this?

This is a difficult one, if you are in the habit of involving your child in outpatient 'post-mortems', eg "Do you think the doctor meant this...?" "Why did they do a scan this time?" etc., then a natural progression should develop in which he gradually begins to take a more prominent role in discussions – and you can then begin to hold back. The next stage perhaps, is to encourage him to go into his consultation on his own, with you joining in at the end. That way your child can make the decision about what to share with you.

It is not the place of this book to dictate timescales but here are some things to consider. Your child may only have a hospital appointment once a year. Because they happen so rarely and are so linked in memory to times when your child was most vulnerable, it is easy to suspend the usual daily rules which we may have already 'signed up to' with our children as they grow older, e.g. allowing them to stay over with friends, respecting their privacy, knocking before entering their bedroom, etc.

If we automatically respect their right to privacy in our home, then shouldn't we also be applying it to hospital appointments etc?

When your child reaches 16, he becomes responsible for signing his own consent form for surgery, or catheterisation. Even with a thoughtfully phased plan of increasing discussion and involvement over several years, it is not easy to prepare your child for this situation.

If he has never been encouraged to take responsibility for his condition, such a situation can be doubly traumatic both for him and for you.

How you can help, is to keep the lines of communication open at all costs. Let him know that you are there to support him at all times, but don't try to "make it better". You can't – and he knows this.

No matter how old your child is when he has to undergo surgery, it is an incredibly difficult time. That feeling of helpless dread does not go away as he gets older.

In many ways you may feel more helpless as your child becomes a young adult because you cannot shoulder his fears and anxieties for him, you cannot "make it better." He has to take some steps alone and all you can do is be there, endlessly patient and prepared to listen to him if he wants to talk, or just be there, if he doesn't.

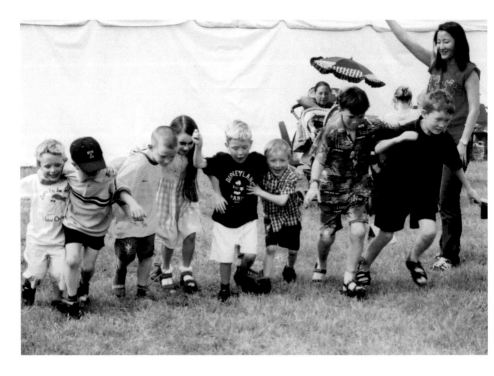

Joining a support group can provide reassurance for patients – and is great fun for the children!

11 FEEDING PROBLEMS
Hints and tips

Generally, babies with heart defects should be treated like healthy babies and fed either by breast or by bottle according to your wishes. You may find though that your baby tires easily while feeding and smaller more frequent feeds may be necessary.

Breast feeding is recommended as breast milk is a complete food and has immunological benefits (i.e., some of the immunities to disease that his mother has are passed on to the baby through the breast milk).

It may be that your baby is separated from you as a newborn because he needs specialist treatment. In this case you can express your milk at four hourly intervals and your milk can be deep frozen and kept for your baby to have. Do not worry if your production of milk seems to diminish during times of stress – continue to express at regular intervals and make sure you drink adequate amounts, then once the baby is able to suck again, the milk supply will increase to meet the baby's demand. (Most hospitals have electric breast pumps and your local National Childbirth Trust may well be able to lend you one for use at home. Most chemists sell hand breast-pumps).

Certain heart defects, which cause the baby to be breathless may mean that your baby is unable to feed either by breast or

bottle initially. If this happens you will find that the nurse will pass a fine tube through the baby's nose down to his stomach and small amounts of milk will be given frequently.

As the baby's condition improves he may be able to take a little of his feed orally either from the breast or the bottle and have the remainder through the tube. Some babies get confused between breast and bottle and are unable to manage both methods. (The sucking technique has to be slightly different!)

In order to estimate how much milk a breast fed baby has taken, he is 'test-weighed'. Before his feed, he is changed and made comfortable, then weighed with all his clothes. The feed is given and he is weighed again with the same clothes and nappy. The number of grammes he has gained is roughly equivalent to the number of millilitres of milk he has drunk.

Sometimes, if a baby finds sucking just too difficult, the feed may be given with a spoon. A small amount of rice-based cereal may be used to thicken the feed slightly.

Your baby may be slower to gain weight than others, but as long as he seems contented and sleeps for reasonable periods, do not worry too much about this. He may require feeding through the night for longer than other babies because he cannot take long feeds, but once he starts sleeping through do not worry about waking him (you need your sleep too). If necessary fit in an extra feed during the day.

If weight gain becomes a real problem and your baby is unable to tolerate extra volume, there are special preparations on the market, which may be added to either breast milk or ordinary infant formula, but do not do this without advice from a dietitian.

If you find that you just cannot cope with breast-feeding do not feel guilty about bottle-feeding. It will not harm your baby to have another milk. Some babies seem to prefer bottle-feeds and some find it easier to suck from a bottle. The important thing is that you and the baby should be as contented as possible!

WEANING YOUR BABY

Solid food may be introduced from about four to six months of age. Start with Baby Rice or mashed banana. Use a small spoon. Do not be tempted to put cereal into the bottle because the baby would have to suck harder. Gradually introduce different foods, but remember that babies do not need extra salt, sugar or other flavourings. (Initially try and avoid wheat-based cereals as there is some evidence that babies can develop malabsorption problems if given wheat too early).

You will find that your baby will establish his own routines and eventually need only three or four feeds a day at normal mealtimes.

Notes 🖉 on feeding

12 SOME GENERAL ADVICE
Answers to questions most parents ask.

1. What *causes* Congenital Heart Disease?

The human heart forms during the first ten weeks of pregnancy and it is during this time that abnormalities occur.

The cause in 90% of cases is unknown. It appears to be a mixture of our complex genetic make-up and some 'trigger' from the environment but the rapid advances in genetic medicine will improve our knowledge and understanding in the future.

It is important to say that it is NO-ONE'S fault. Some factors, however, are known, e.g. when the heart is involved in general chromosomal abnormalities such as Down's syndrome or a gene problem such as Marfan's syndrome. Occasionally the heart maybe damaged by an infection such as German measles, or by drugs, some anti convulsants or excess alcohol.

2. Should immunisations be given?

All routine immunisations should be given against diphtheria, tetanus, whooping cough, polio, HIB, meningococcus, measles, mumps, rubella. BCG is also important if indicated. The incidence of these infections has reduced dramatically as a result of these immunisation programmes. Whooping cough can be a very serious illness in children with heart problems, and unless there is a definite contra-indication, the child should be protected by being immunised.

3. Infections – how do they affect my child?

Infections should be treated as in the normal child. Blue children when they have a high temperature require lots to drink to prevent dehydration which may further thicken their abnormally thick blood.

If vomiting is a significant problem then it is important to call your doctor.

4. What about education and going to school?

The majority of children are able to attend normal schools, and can join in all normal activities. Children, who are significantly 'blue' (cyanosed) tolerate cold weather poorly, and special arrangements can be made to avoid school playgrounds in inclement weather.

Those who are significantly breathless should be allowed to rest when they become tired. The children usually set their own limits far better than anyone else. In senior school, there are a few heart conditions in which competitive sports, such as judo, rowing and karate should be avoided. These are significant aortic stenosis, pulmonary hypertension and hypertrophic cardiomyopathy.

Reasonable exercise and swimming, however, should be encouraged.

5. Dental care – is any special treatment needed?

YES. You MUST Tell your dentist that your child has a congenital heart disorder.

It is known that patients who have bad dental hygiene with lots of caries and unhealthy gums force bacteria into their blood stream with chewing and biting. Cardiac teams strongly recommend regular attention to dental care, the use of fluoride toothpaste – and possibly, fluoride drops, if there is no fluoride in the local water. The amount of fluoride in your local tap water can be ascertained by contacting your local Community Health Service Office. Dental treatment involving extractions, scaling, polishing, and deep fillings, requires your child to be given a large dose of antibiotic an hour before the dental work. This is because these proce-dures are known to produce bacteria in the blood stream. Many children with heart disease will need this prophylactic antibiotic therapy for the rest of their lives.

Small children with heart problems often require many medications that contain large amounts of sugar to make them palatable. Prevention of dental caries and bad gums is more difficult in our group of children.

Some useful tips are:

a) Avoid sugary foods and drinks between meals or last thing at night.

b) Teeth should be cleaned after medicines, and particularly so after the night time dose. Ask your doctor if tablets can be used rather than medicines.

Ask if sugar free medicines are available.

c) Get your child into the habit of regular toothbrushing at an early age.

d) Use fluoride toothpaste. Think about added fluoride drops.

e) Plan to start visits to the dentist from an early age even if it is only to accompany you so that he is used to going.

6. Is any special care needed with travelling and holidays?

The majority of patients have no difficulties with air or sea flights.

Do ensure that adequate medications are taken abroad. Avoid too much exposure to sun and ensure your child does not get dehydated, particularly in small children and those who are 'blue'. If your child is very blue or breathless, discuss your plans with your doctors. They may well advise you to inform your travel agent and the airline so that arrangements can be made for oxygen to be available during the flight and a wheelchair, if needed.

It is important to remember that although the cabins are pressurised on all flights, this is equivalent to a height of 5000 feet (1600 metres). This is equivalent to breathing at the top of Ben Nevis and produces a fall in oxygen saturation of about 4%. Most children will cope very well with this. Don't forget to allow enough time for these arrangements to be made if necessary.

7. Insurance: Are there any special conditions?

Life insurance may be difficult and an excess premium may be demanded. There may be some difficulty in getting insurance cover for mortgages. The advice is to shop around.

There is *usually* no difficulty with travel

insurance, but you may require a letter from your doctor saying that your child is stable and no particular complication is expected.

Personal and property insurance cause no problems.

8. Smoking: what effect does it have?

Smoking produces damage to the normally smooth lining of the arteries. Clots form on this now roughened area. It is the blockage of arteries as a result of these clots that produce heart attacks and strokes. In addition, smoking produces chronic chest infections and cancer of the lung, gullet and mouth. Patients with congenital heart problems are likely to be at greater risk from smoking than the average person. Children **are much more likely to smoke** if their parents smoke. Passive smoking, that is regular breathing in other peoples exhaled smoke, causes similar problems to smoking itself.

SMOKING IS BAD FOR US ALL .
It is the biggest avoidable health hazard in the developed world.

9. What about alcoholic drinks?

Small amounts cause no problem in adults. Excess consumption of alcoholic drinks is harmful and may lead to emotional and behavioural problems. It can be linked to many accidents in adults and adolescents. It is important for you to set your "heart" child a good example by sensible consumption of alcoholic drinks in the family.

EXCESS ALCOHOL CONSUMPTION
is the second largest avoidable hazard in developed countries.

10 Diet: how important is 'eating healthily?'

A good balanced diet is especially important for children with heart problems. Babies and small children require fat to grow at a normal rate, and also to supply essential vitamins. But in older children and adolescents, it is important to avoid too much fat, particularly animal saturated fats and too much salt and sugar. Many of the manufactured so-called 'convenience' foods in our supermarkets are packed with salt, sugar, animal fat, preservatives and chemicals for flavouring and colour.

It is better to cook with fresh natural or organic ingredients if you can.

Try to eat wholemeal bread, wholewheat cereals, vegetables, pulses (i.e. peas and beans) fruit, fish, relatively lean meat and polyunsaturated fats. Try not to add excess salt at the table. A little salt in cooking, however, is acceptable. Avoid greasy fast foods. Grilled shish kebabs and salads are better for you than burgers and shop fish and chips, although the occasional treat will do you no harm, unless you have been given medical advice to the contrary.

Further practical advice on diet can be found in 3 useful booklets published by the Health Education Authority, entitled:

Guide to Healthy Eating, Exercise. Why Bother? and Do You Take Sugar?

See Chapter 16 for more information.

11. Weight – does it affect health?

Obesity (excess weight) in the adolescent and adult causes more work for the heart to do. The fatter you are, the more likely you are to have a high blood pressure, develop late-onset diabetes damaging heart muscle and artery walls. Avoid being too thin as this is bad for you also. Aim for the average weight for your age and height. This is specially important for "heart" children

12. Driving: are there any problems for young people with heart problems?

Usually there are none unless there is a risk of sudden collapse, which is very rare. Patients who have pacemakers inserted can hold a regular driving licence, but are unable to hold a heavy goods vehicle or PCV licence. DVLA driving licence application forms ask various medical questions. As you are legally required to provide correct information, ask your GP or cardiac specialist if you are in any doubt. It is better for aspiring young drivers to seek advice than risk the possibilty of finding their insurance is invalid due to some technicality.

13. Contraception: is there any special advice for young adults?

Usually, normal contraceptive practices involving the low dose combined pill can be used in the majority of post-operative patients, and those with minor problems whose hearts are functionally good, for example – small holes, mild to moderate valve problems. The exceptions, however, are:

a) those patients who have thick blood (called polycythaemia), usually as a result of being blue.

b) high blood pressure in either the lung or the body artery.

c) those with sluggish circulation either from weak heart muscle or from a Fontan-type operation connecting the right atrium or the veins directly into the lung artery.

d) those on anticoagulants.

Their management needs to be discussed carefully. Sometimes, the very low dose mini-pills can be used. In others, the prog-esterone only pill, injectable Depo-provera or barrier/sheath methods are suggested.

Interuterine coils are not usually suitable for young women but if used, need antibiotic prophylaxis for insertion and removal. Ask your doctor for advice early! Emergency 'morning after' pills are usually acceptable. Unwanted pregnancies are to be avoided.

14. Pregnancy and Delivery

If there is little in the way of symptoms, then pregnancy is very well tolerated. If the patient is breathless, regular supervision will be required, often requiring extra periods of rest, particularly towards the end of pregnancy. The delivery almost certainly will need to be in hospital. If blueness is a problem, there is a higher incidence of miscarriage. Pregnancy is known to be unwise in those patients who are very cyanosed and in those who have a very high blood pressure in the lung artery.

> **For more general information about pregnancy, see the very clearly written 'Pregnancy Book' from the Health Education Authority**

15. What risk do we stand of further children with congenital heart problems?

The chance of any child being born with a heart problem is approximately 1%. If there is already one child in the family with such a problem, then the risks that a further heart problem will occur in that family rise to approximately 3%. This means that the chance of a normal child from the point of view of the heart is 97%. If there are two children affected, the chances of further heart problems rise to 10%, if three children are affected in the family the risks rise to approximately 25%. Generally, the type of defect running within one family is similar.

16. Antenatal Scan

Antenatal diagnosis is possible by use of special ultrasound equipment and skills. Routine anomaly scans are now undertaken around 16-20 weeks to look at the whole of the developing baby. Images of the heart can frequently be seen, normally occupying a third of the diameter of the chest, there being an equal balance between both sides of the heart and four chambers with two filling valves normally visualised. It may also be possible to see more complex problems on routine scans.

If there is a concern about this routine scan or the family is at a somewhat higher risk than the average family for having a baby with a heart problem, for example, those with previous children with heart problems or diabetic mothers, then a more detailed scan focusing solely on the heart would be proposed. This may be undertaken in the local hospital or may need referral to a unit often linked to a paediatric cardiac unit.

17. What are the risks that offspring will have a heart problem?

It is likely that the children of patients who themselves have congenital heart problems will have an approximately 5% chance of having a heart problem. It appears that the risks are slightly higher if the mother, rather than the father, has the heart problem. There is no increased risk to the children of normal brothers and sisters in a family where one child has heart disease.

18. Employment: what jobs aren't suitable?

The good news is, that with suitable encouragement from parents and carers, the majority of patients can undertake almost any job.

The exceptions are the armed forces who are currently very reluctant to take anyone with a heart problem, even if minor or if successfully corrected. Heavy manual work, however, may not be ideal if there is a long standing reduction in cardiac efficiency.

13 MEDICINES
Drugs used to treat heart problems & what they do.

Many children will not require medicines at all. Medicines are often known by two names, the chemical or generic name which is the official one, and proprietary or brand names of the companies who market them, of which there may be several. Some children will require one or more of the medicines described below:

1. DIGOXIN

This increases the force of contraction of the heart muscle and in addition slows down conduction within the electrical system. It is used when the heart muscle needs extra support, and also in the treatment of fast heart rates.

Nausea and reduced appetite may occur as side-effects if the patient is rather sensitive to it.

2. FRUSEMIDE & CHLOROTHIAZIDE

These are diuretics which make the kidneys pass more urine. The children lose sodium, chloride, potassium and water. When the heart is not working very well, water and salt accumulate in the body, liver and lungs, making particularly the lungs rather heavy. When these drugs are given, the lungs become somewhat lighter, easier to expand and, less energy is used in breathing. Try to avoid excess salt when taking these drugs as this reduces their efficiency.

3. SPIRONOLACTONE & AMILORIDE

These are weaker diuretics which hold on to potassium. They are often used in conjunction with the other diuretics.

4. POTASSIUM SUPPLEMENTS

Some duretics make the patient lose potassium, a chemical essential to the body.

These supplements are used to replace the loss and are used in association with diuretics. They are, unfortunately, rather unpalatable. Natural replacements in the form of orange juice, tomato juice and bananas may be used instead.

5. HYDRALAZINE, CAPTOPRIL & ENALAPRIL ETC.

These drugs dilate blood vessels and as a result reduce blood pressure. They can be used in patients with high blood pressure to reduce it to normal. They can also be used in those patients with a normal blood pressure and a weak heart. By reducing the blood pressure this reduces the work of the heart.

6. PROPRANOLOL

This is a beta blocker that reduces the rate and force of contraction in the heart muscle. It is useful in treating fast heart rates, high blood pressure and also relieving spasm of heart muscle in tetralogy of Fallot. Similar drugs are now being used in the treatment of heart failure.

7. ANTIARRHYTHMIC DRUGS

Are used to control tachycardias – fast heart beats – and include Verapamil, Disopyramide, Lignocaine, Mexilitene, Flecainide, Amiodarone, Adenosine and beta blockers.

8. ANTICOAGULANTS

Children who have artificial valves made of metal and plastic require blood thinning medicines in the form of Warfarin to prevent clots developing on the valve. Regular blood tests are required to assess the level of thinning of blood. Your child will be given a card on which are recorded the Warfarin dosage and the result of the blood test. Aspirin and Dipyridamole are sometimes used to prevent the blood platelets sticking together post-operatively. Anticoagulants are often used in adolescent patients with large weak hearts, and also those with high blood pressure in the lung arteries.

9. SEDATIVES

Children with heart problems are sometimes very fractious and mild sedation, for example Trichloryl is often very helpful in allaying anxiety and ensuring adequate rest for the child.

10. ANTIBIOTICS

A whole armoury of drugs which are used to fight infection in the same way as for a child with a normal heart, and especially to prevent endocarditis during interventional procedures.

11. INTRAVENOUS DRUGS

Very strong medications can be given directly via a vein (intravenously) to improve the circulation to the body and to the lungs. Examples of these are Dopamine, Adrenaline, Nitroprusside, Prostaglandin, Prostacyclin and Tolazoline.

12. PARACETAMOL

Generally speaking, it is safe to give your child paracetamol if he has a temperature. Give the dose recommended on the box for your child's age.

TAKING MEDICINES

When you are given a new medicine please check you know the answers to the following questions:

a) Its name.
b) The reason for taking it.
c) How often during the day it should be taken – and its relation to meals.
d) For how long?
e) Does it upset any other medicines?
f) What, if any, are the side effects that might be expected?

GIVING MEDICINES TO YOUR BABY

This can be a difficult task but obviously it is important that the baby receives the right amount of drug at the right time.

Make sure that you understand the instructions on the bottle. Give the medicine before the feed. Use a spoon, a small syringe or medicine glass (an egg cup would do). Hold the baby firmly with his head slightly back and give not more than a third of a teaspoonful in his mouth at once. You will find that the baby will get used to the strange taste of the medicine. Do not be tempted to put medicines into your baby's bottle. This would make the milk taste strange and may have the effect of putting the baby off his feeds. If your baby is sick immediately after the medicine is given, wait a while and then repeat it. Do not repeat if there is an interval of 15-20 minutes because some drugs are absorbed quite quickly from the stomach. If vomiting is a frequent occurrence, consult your doctor.

Antibiotics are usually made up in a syrupy substance so if your older child has to have these, follow the medicine with a drink of water to clean the syrup off the teeth.

14 STATE BENEFITS AND SUPPORT SERVICES

Benefits and the rates at which benefits are paid are constantly changing. Therefore in this chapter we will aim to summarise and signpost you to main benefits payable in relation to having a sick child. It is for this reason also that we have not listed rates payable. These and other information, as well as packs for claiming benefits are available from several different sources.

A main source is the **Benefits Agency**, whose local offices are listed in your phone book.

The Benefits Agency also runs several inquiry lines including the *Benefit Enquiry Line* for people with disabilities, this number is: **0800 88 22 00**. The central helpline number for child benefits is: **08701 55 55 40**.

Contact a Family(CaF) publish a factsheet *Child Disability Benefits and other Sources of Help* which you can receive by calling the CaF Freephone Helpline 0808 808 3555, or visit their web site *www.cafamily.org.uk*.

Other agencies where you can obtain information about benefits available are larger Post Offices, Citizens Advice Bureaux and Social Services.

DISABILITY LIVING ALLOWANCE (DLA)

This is a benefit for people who have a mental or physical illness or disability. You can claim DLA if you are under 65. It can be paid on top of other benefits and does not reduce the amount you get. DLA has 2 parts

– one part is based on care needs and the other on mobility needs. The **Care Part** is paid at 3 different levels and the **Mobility Part** at 2 levels. You can receive one level for the Care Part and one level for the Mobility Part, both being based on an assessment of your child's needs.

A child can qualify for the Care Part of DLA from birth and be paid from the age of 3 months. If the child is terminally ill it can be paid from birth. The Mobility Part can only be paid from three years from April 2001.

For the Care Part and the lowest rate of the Mobility Part of DLA, children under the age of 16 have to show their needs are greater than those of a child of the same age who has no disability.

You can receive an application pack from sources listed above. When filling out the form, think carefully about how much you have to do for your child. Considerable weight is given to the extra amount of supervision that needs to be provided for a claimant. Therefore it is helpful to think about the extra amount of time you have to spend supervising your child and why. Ask yourself what tasks you have to do for him at a particular age that are not required for other children.

Examples are: tasks that may be related to the medication your child has to take, or the assistance he needs with dressing if he tires very easily.

The Care Part The level of payment your child receives will depend on the extra level of "supervision" he requires. "Supervision" may be needed because he has a physical or learning disability where he maybe confused or forgetful, or have falls or fits, or sometimes needs urgent medical help.

The Mobility Part – He qualifies for the *higher rate* if he is virtually unable to walk or can only walk with severe discomfort e.g. pain or breathlessness.

If your car is used for the sole purpose of transporting your disabled child you will also qualify for road tax exemption. If you think you may qualify for road tax exemption write to the **Mobility Allowance** Unit from where your payment book comes. Your child qualifies for the *lower rate* if he needs guidance or supervision when walking outdoors, in unfamiliar places, or he has falls or fits.

To apply for DLA telephone **0800 88 22 00** and ask for a *DLA Claim Pack* – **Form DLA1**.(NB. for children under 16, ask for Form **DLA1 Child**). Your claim, if granted, will be eligible from the time that you asked for the form from the DSS.

FAMILIES AND BENEFITS

Here is a list of the main social security benefits to which families may be entitled:

1. Child Benefit – for children under 16, or under 19 in full-time education;

2. Working Families Tax Credit (WFTC) – for families or lone parents on low incomes where one partner is working at least 16 hours a week; this replaced family credit in October 1999. (WFTC now includes a credit to meet the cost of childcare. You can get a credit worth 70% of eligible childcare costs to a specified limit.)

3. Income Support – for families or lone parents who do not have to be available for work. If you, or someone for whom you claim, receives Income Support, you may also be eligible for the following:

4. Jobseekers allowance – for families or lone parents who do not have to be available for work;

5. Housing Benefit – for help with rent;

6. Council Tax Benefit and council tax reductions – for help with council tax;

7. Education Benefits – for help with school uniforms, minor awards and free school meals;

8. Social Fund – grants and loans to meet the cost of "one -off" items; this includes cold weather payments for weeks of severe cold weather if you have a disabled child, or a child under 5. This benefit will be automatically paid if you receive income support.

9. Health Benefits – help with costs of prescriptions, dental treatment, sight tests, glasses, fares to hospital, milk and vitamins.

BENEFITS FOR PEOPLE WITH A DISABILITY WHO START WORK

Severe Disablement Allowance (SDA) & **Incapacity Benefit (ICB)**

You get Incapacity Benefit (ICB) if you are incapable of work and have paid enough national insurance contributions. You get Severe Disablement Allowance (SDA) if you are incapable of work but have not paid enough national insurance contributions. You can get this benefit from your 16th birthday if you cannot work. SDA can be paid to you whilst you are in special education (school or college) and you still get it when you leave, if you are unable to work. However Child Benefit is not payable if you get SDA.

Most 16 and 17 year olds cannot get means-tested benefits. Young people are expected either to be supported by parents, or be in education, full time employment or Youth Training. Income Support is only paid to people who don't have to sign-on as unemployed, e.g. those who are unfit for work. Therefore, if you cannot work and you meet the usual rules for getting income support (e.g £8,000 or less in savings and not working for more than 16 hours a week) you may be able to claim in your own right while you are 16 or 17 if you are;

- disabled and still at school or college;

- not at school or college and the Benefits Agency accept you as being incapable of work due to illness or disability

PASSPORT TO OTHER BENEFITS

If you get Income Support you can also get;

- **free** NHS prescriptions

- **free** NHS dental treatment:

- **free** eye test and vouchers towards the cost of glasses;

- **free** travel to hospital for NHS treatment if you produce proof that you are in receipt of any of these benefits: Income Support, Family Credit, Income-based Jobseekers Allowance or Disabled Person's Tax Credit and you are escorting your child to and from hospital for NHS treatment, your fares can be refunded, usually at outpatients clinic or transport office).

- access to grants and loans from the Social Fund.

INVALID CARE ALLOWANCE

Invalid Care Allowance (ICA) is a weekly benefit you can get if you are looking after a disabled person/child for at least 35 hours a week. The disabled person/child must be receiving certain rates of disability living allowance. It is important to remember though, that you cannot get ICA if you are getting at least the same amount from: Jobseeker's Allowance, Retirement Pension, Maternity Allowance, Widow's Benefit, Incapacity Benefit or Severe Disablement Allowance. Even if you cannot get ICA because you get another benefit instead, it may be worth claiming it, as you may qualify for an extra benefit, a Carer's Premium,which will be paid over and above your Income Support, or Income-Based Jobseeker's Allowance.

Leaflet NI196 Social Security Benefit Rates provides up to date benefit rates, earnings rules etc.

Copies of these are available from your local DSS office or from the HeartLine office (See Chapter 17, page 111 for address).

The Child Poverty Action Group,
94 White Lion Street, London N1 9PF.
Tel: 020 7837 7979
Fax: 020 7837 6414
Email: staff@cpag.org.uk
www.cpag.org.uk

CPAG produces excellent publications on welfare rights and benefits. These are also available at libraries. CPAG also run an advice service for professionals which is not open to the public.

Copies of these books are also available at the HeartLine office. They can help you find your way around the State Benefit System and are not difficult to understand.

OTHER FINANCIAL SUPPORT

People on Income Support or a low income can sometimes get additional help from various organisations for specific things e.g. help with hospital expenses, help to buy a spin dryer, or to have a holiday if they have a sick child, or are themselves disabled, or for any reason where the stress in the family can be judged to be greater than average.

Various associations help in situations like this, for example, the Chest, Heart and Stroke Association or the Family Fund for sick and disabled children. Apply to the former through a health visitor or social worker. The latter you can contact directly yourself. The Fund will usually send their own Social Worker to assess your individual needs. They are sympathetic towards help required for driving lessons e.g. to get your child to and from hospital, doctors etc., the installation of telephones, or providing for specific needs of that child including help with holidays.

Some professions, like the Armed Forces, the Civil Service and several others, have their own funds and will consider applications from families. You can apply directly to the funds themselves, or ask your health visitor or social worker to apply.

The Citizens Advice Bureau may be able to give you advice about local trusts. Sometimes Public Libraries also have information about local charities. Lions Clubs and Rotary Clubs might also give families help.

TRAVEL

Trains – A registered disabled person may get half price travel for himself and one accompanying adult if he has a Railcard. Ask at your local station for information.

Taxis – If you live in London and receive Mobility Allowance, or your doctor certifies by letter that you or your child are unable to use public transport because of a disability that seriously affects your walking ability, you can get a **Taxicard** which enables you to make a journey of up to £9, in the Greater London Area for only £1.25. Ask your Post Office for a form. Your hospital's social services department should also keep these forms.

RADAR – Royal Association for Disability and Rehabilitation provides information about discounts and concessions on cars for disabled people and have a range of useful fact sheets on transport and mobility issues.

'Door to Door' This guide provides transport information for people with disabilities. Originally published by the Department of Transport Mobility Unit, it has recently been updated and is now available through RADAR at £8 including p & p.

Contact address:
RADAR, 12 City Forum,
250 City Road,
London EC1V 8AF
Tel: 020 7250 3222
www.@radar.org.uk

Other practical information:

THE FAMILY

Your family may be under a lot of stress if your child is ill. Remember that it might help to talk to your health visitor or GP. You could also contact your local social services department. The Children and Families practice group may have a social worker specifically for families with children with special needs Alternatively, it maybe possible for them to refer you to a voluntary organisation like Homestart who provide trained volunteers to befriend families with children under five years who are under particular stress and do not have family support systems available.

Social Services can sometimes arrange for a Home Help to come to the house on a short term basis when the family is in the middle of a crisis and is finding it difficult to cope. Alternatively they can supply you with a list of registered care agencies and child-minders who are able to provide extra help. They may also know of any local parent support groups.

Community workers, like social workers and health visitors, will also know of any special playgroups or nurseries or other facilities that might be available for a child with a heart condition, to help the child and to relieve the other members of the family from this extra stress.

WORK

If a child goes into hospital, sometimes a father may have to take time off work to help take care of the rest of the family, or may be in hospital with the child. While some employers are sympathetic and grant compassionate leave, others may be less understanding and fathers may end up receiving no pay.

It may well help to get the hospital social worker to contact your work and discuss the problem with them: sometimes employers really do not realise the implications of long term hospital stays or repeated outpatient appointments.

However, if no pay is granted, parents may then need advice and help about applying for Income Support. Self-employed fathers are particularly vulnerable in this situation and may well find that the benefit they receive is small. Consult your hospital social worker for advice about this.

STATE HOUSING

Sometimes home conditions are such that they are detrimental to the child:

eg: there are a lot of stairs and no lift and the child's condition limits his physical ability, or the accommodation is damp and/or there is inadequate heating. Generally, in situations like this, a medical letter can be sent to the Housing Department supporting a housing transfer request. This may speed things up but the response you get will vary greatly from area to area according to local resources.

HOUSING ALTERATIONS

If alterations are made to your home to assist your disabled child, e.g. installations of showers, downstairs lavatories, alterations for wheelchairs etc: you may be eligible for a grant for this work, depending the area where you live. Contact your Occupational Therapist at your local Social Services Department for information before you start work. If adaptations have been made to a house to make it more accessible for a disabled child, you maybe eligible for a reduction in council tax, again, depending on your local authority's rules.

PUSHCHAIRS and BUGGIES

If your child's heart condition limits mobility considerably, as he gets bigger you may need a larger, strong pushchair or buggy to get about. If he is aged two and a half years or more, you should be able to get a buggy or wheelchair for him from your local Wheelchair Service Centre. Since 1996, powered outdoor/indoor wheelchairs can be provided for severely disabled people, if they are unable to walk or propel a manual wheelchair. Each area has its own criteria. Some centres will provide a double buggy if you have a younger child not yet walking as well as a disabled child who needs assistance with walking. Your GP, health visitor, District Health Authority or hospital should also be able to give you information on this.

ORANGE BADGE SCHEME

A disabled family member entitles you to park your car in disabled parking bays. Contact your Social Services Department about applying for an orange badge.

WORK FOR YOUNG ADULTS

If your child has left school and wants to start to look for work and is registered as disabled, contact the DRO (Disablement Resettlement Officer) at your local Job Centre.

SIGNING-ON RULES

It might be useful for parents to know when signing on for work, rules for the unemployed can be waived at the discretion of the Benefit Officer.

This is waived in special circumstances e.g. if a parent is staying in hospital away from home with a child who is temporarily ill, and either the other parent who normally looks after the child is unable to do so, or if there is no other parent.

This regulation comes under Supplementary Benefit Conditions of the Entitlement Regulations 1981 No 1525 Regulation 6.

EDUCATION

The 1981 Education Act states that all school age children have a right to education and therefore it is the statutory duty of the Education Authorities to see that they receive it.

Sometimes education really is a problem, if the child is too unwell to go to school, or physically unable to cope with the journey or move about school. It can be difficult if the school is large, on several different levels or your child has to go out of doors to get to some classrooms. These things are worth checking before he begins at a new school. With a little imagination it may be possible to juggle the school timetable slightly so that a child with a heart problem, or indeed any physical disability, does not have to expend energy needlessly to reach classrooms spaced a long way apart. After surgery, a child may have a period of time away from school and it may be necessary to arrange home tuition. If you think this is going to be necessary, get in touch with your local Education Department in plenty of time as these things do take a while to sort out.

Use this space to jot down any personal notes on benefits:

15 BEREAVEMENT

At some time in the lives of children with severe heart defects, most have periods of being 'on the critical list'. For the majority, these periods are mercifully short-lived and the trauma quickly forgotten in the happiness of recovery. There are occasions however, when children die. This is devastating for the parents and relatives and deeply upsetting for the medical/nursing team, who expend so much effort in prolonging life. When a child remains critically ill, no-one knows exactly what to do or say.

Many parents in this situation are aware of feeling alienated from nursing staff and other parents in the unit. They desperately want to know exactly what is happening to their child but are terrified of hearing the worst. Staff tend, to some extent, to follow the lead given by the parents and so develop what, to some parents, seems to amount to a conspiracy of silence.

There is no completely satisfactory way of overcoming this problem.

Death is not a subject which we in western society are encouraged to discuss. Parents may be afraid of appearing morbid if they ask if their child is going to die, and medical staff hesitate to bring it up for fear of upsetting the parents. At the same time it is the one thing which is on everyone's minds. Not being able to voice this almost immobilising fear adds to the strain. Many parent also feel that they cannot mention the word 'dying' when their child is still fighting to live.

The grief which occurs as a result of bereavement has been described as 'a reaction in which normal functioning no longer holds'. In fact, many bereaved parents talk of feeling as though 'they are going mad', they worry about coping with the intensity of their feelings and find the rapid changes which their emotions go through, very bewildering.

If you have suffered a bereavement, or you are supporting parents who have, this chapter has been written in the hope that it may help for you to know that these swinging changes in mood are normal. Unless a parent has been through the loss of a child of their own, they cannot fully understand what you are going through.

One of the worst aspects of loss that parents describe is the total inability to do anything about what has happened. Most things that occur in our lives we have some control over, or we can do something to ease the situation. There is nothing one can do to change the death of a child. Often it is the sense of helplessness that this knowledge brings that adds to feelings of anger and pain.

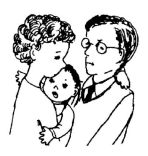

THE PROCESS OF GRIEVING

It is generally believed that there are three main stages of grief, and that these have to be worked through – but the order and timing of each part of the stages does vary with each individual.

Briefly, the stages are: **shock and numbness**, these are the **initial** reactions to loss and may include actual physical symptoms of palpitations, muscular weakness or nausea. The numbness makes our surroundings seem unreal and remote, as though we are distanced from what is happening. Another aspect of this first stage is a denial of what has happened. Parents temporarily 'forget' their loss and find themselves laying their child's place at the table for example, running their bath or buying an item of clothing while out shopping. This temporary denial of reality is also perfectly normal.

The second stage is a gradual realisation of what has happened and this is accompanied by rapidly changing feelings of anger, apathy, exhaustion, grief and guilt. Parents may want to withdraw from the outside world, or they may find themselves involved in sudden bursts of activity.

The third stage is a gradual realisation that you are able to accept memories without overwhelming grief and you are able to resume forming plans for your future. Decisions become easier to make and practical problems are more easily dealt with.

These stages do vary with each individual and it is impossible to put a time-scale on them. The very fact that they do vary, can create pressures for a couple grieving the loss of their child. If one partner is still in the first stage of numbness and disbelief and the other is experiencing overwhelming feelings of anger and despair their emotions and reactions are at odds. They find it difficult to express what they are feeling for fear of hurting one another, and this at a time when each most needs the support of the other. During these times it may help if both partners have another listener outside the immediate family circle to whom they can voice the feelings they are experiencing.

SOME ADVICE FOR HELPERS

It is not easy for parents to start rebuilding their lives after the death of their child. Relatives and friends who offered support in the beginning may drift away, thinking that the worst is over. And the parents are left feeling isolated and depressed because they are still mourning their loss. Often when they need to talk about their child and the way they feel, others may turn away, embarrassed to talk about the dead.

There are some DOs and DON'Ts drawn up by the Compassionate Friends which help those who know bereaved parents. They suggest that you let your concern and caring show and that you are available – to listen, run errands, help with the children or whatever else seems needed at the time.

... ***Do*** say you are sorry about what happened to their child and about their pain and allow them to express as much grief as they are feeling at that moment and are willing to share.

... ***Do*** encourage them to be patient with themselves and not to expect too much and allow them to talk about the child they have lost as much and as often as they want to.

... *Do* talk about the special qualities of that child and give extra attention to brothers or sisters (they too are hurt and confused and in need of attention which their parents may not be able to give at this time).

... *Do* reassure the parents that they did everything they could, and tell them of everything true and positive about the care given to their child.

... *Don't* avoid the parents because you are uncomfortable, (being avoided by friends adds pain to an already intolerably painful experience).

... *Don't* say you know how they feel (have you lost a child?), or tell them what they should feel or do – like saying 'You ought to be feeling better now' or 'You must pull yourself together'.

...*Don't* change the subject when they mention their dead child or avoid mentioning their child's name because you are scared to remind them of their pain (they will not have forgotten it).

... *Don't* try to find something positive about the death or suggest they can have another child (it would not replace the one they have lost).

... *Don't* make any comments which in any way suggest that the care given to their child at home, in hospital or wherever was inadequate (parents are plagued by feelings of doubt and guilt without any help from their family and friends).

Finally... *Don't* let your own sense of helplessness keep you from reaching out to a bereaved parent. No matter how hard it may seem to you, do remember that what they are going through is so much worse and the knowledge that you do care and are concerned will help them much more than silence.

CARE FROM THE HOSPITAL

Many Cardiac Units are becoming increasingly concerned about providing some form of ongoing support for bereaved parents and make a point of inviting parents back to talk over with staff what happened to their child. Some parents welcome this, as at the time of their child's death, there may be too much numbness and sadness to think about why their child died.

Later, however, the questions may start and they need to be answered. For many parents too, the staff who cared for their child may be their last link with him and because of this they may want to go back to the unit. Equally though they need a reason for doing so. Obviously this is a very personal decision but it is important that parents do know the choice exists. If bereaved parents are not aware of this, or have not had contact with the unit since, it may be helpful to contact the ward sister, or a member of staff they were close to during their child's time in the unit, and ask if a visit can be arranged.

Many families find coming back to discuss their child's illness and death with senior members of the team helpful. The optimum time for this visit varies from family to family and is often around six weeks after the child's death. If you have not heard from the team involved then get in touch.

CHAPTER 16 RECOMMENDED READING LIST

Sources of further information

Books for children

1. GOING TO THE DOCTOR OR HOSPITAL

a) *Going to the Hospital*
by Anne Civardi. Usborne, 1986

b) *Why am I going to hospital?*
by Carole Livingston
Angus & Robertson, 1983

Suitable for 5+ age group. A lively, down to earth description of why a child may go to hospital and the sorts of things that will occur. For example, X-ray, blood tests etc.

c) Topsy and Tim go to Hospital
by Jean & Gareth Adamson
Ladybird, 1988

School and pre-school age. A good introduction to hospital for young patients and their brothers and sisters.

d) *Spot's Hospital Visit*
by Eric Hall, William Heinemann 1987

e) I don't want to go to Hospital
by Bernard Stone, Andersen Press, 1994

An enjoyable story about a little princess who doesn't want to go to hospital but when she finally does, enjoys herself so much she wants to go back again.

f) Emergency Mouse by Bernard Stone
Arrow Books, 1994

School and pre-school age. Anaesthetic, operation and recovery are covered.

2. ABOUT THE HEART

The Heart for Children
Franklin Watts, 1983
The Heart and Human Body Series
Suitable for 11+ age group.

For older children who want to understand how the heart works so that they have a better idea of their own problem.

3. BEREAVEMENT
Material to help children

These and other books are available through The Librarian, The Compassionate Friends, 77 Rectory Lane, Leybourne, West Malling, Kent ME19 5HD.

a) *Badger's Parting Gift*
by Susan Varley, Lion Books 1992

b) *Beginnings and endings, with lifetimes in between*, Dragons World, 1983.

c) *Waterbugs and Dragonflies*
by Doris Stickney, Cassell, 1989

d) *Charlotte's Web*, by E B White
Penguin Puffin Books, 1973

Animal story including chapter dealing with death of the heroine.

e) *Watership Down*, by Richard Adams
Penguin Puffin Books, 1973

Animal story ending with deaths of the heroes.

The following are available through the Child Bereavement Trust, telephone 0845 3571000:

f) *Someone Died*, (Video)
   It happened to me (and Pack:)
These help children and young people to explore and find expression for their feelings.

g) *Memory Box and Memory Wallet*
For keeping things that are the reminders of the child who died.

Books for adults

4. GENERAL

a) *Surgery and your Heart*
   by D Ross & B Hyams
   Beaconsfield Publishers 1982
This book was written for the layman in order that the patient or parents, the family and the medical team can get together on common ground.

b) *A Guide to Grants for Individuals in Need*
By Sarah Harland and Dave Griffiths, available from the Directory of Social Change www.dsc.org.uk/bookshop 7th Edition 2000/2001. Contains details of over 2,300 national and local trusts which make grants to individuals.

c) *Choosing for Children*
   by Priscilla Alderson
   Oxford University Press, 1990
A book which looks at Cardiac Units through parents eyes and explores the subject of informed consent.

d) *Contraception – Your Questions Answered* by John Guillebaud
   Oxford University Press

5. HEALTH GUIDANCE

a) Guide to Healthy Eating
   Exercise, Why Bother?
   Do You Take Sugar?
   Health Education Authority
Three excellent booklets on healthy diet. from The Health Education Authority, Hamilton House, Mabledon Place, London WC1H 9JX at about 10p each.

b) *The Pregnancy Book*
   Health Education Authority
Another very clearly written manual published by the Health Education Authority at about 50p, but available free of charge from maternity units for first-time mothers.

6. BEREAVEMENT
Material to help adults
These books and videos are available through the Child Bereavement Trust, telephone 01494 446648:

a) *The CBT Information Pack*
This contains valuable information for parents and professional alike - anyone who is involved or concerned with grieving families following the death of a baby or child, or when a child is bereaved.

b) *When our Baby Died (Video)*
Parents describe what it has meant to them, how it has changed their lives, how they have mourned and found support for themselves.

c) *Grieving after the Death of your Baby*
A book about grief after the death of a baby through miscarriage or perinatal death.

b) *When a Child Grieves (Video)*
Double video for parents when a family or child is bereaved.

Tapes: The Loss of a Baby
e) Tape 1: *Death of Your Baby*;
f) Tape 2: *Stillbirth and Neonatal Death*
In Urdu and English.

g) *Memory Box and Memory Wallet*
For keeping the special things that are the reminders of the child who died.

h) The following leaflets are available from The Compassionate Friends telephone 0117 966 5202:
- Preparing your child's funeral
- A father's grief
- Grieving Couples
- A mother's grief
- Childless parents
- Teenagers
- To bereaved grandparents
- Helping younger brothers and sisters
- The bereaved parent coping alone
- On inquests (England and Wales)

i) The following websites may be helpful:

- www.grannyg.bc.ca/ckidbook/grief
- www.childbereavement.org.uk
- www.tcf.org.uk
- www.inspirit.com.au/books

j) *The Courage to Grieve*
by Judy Tatelman, Heinnemen, 1981
A guide through the emotions of grief.

k) *A Grief Observed*, by C S Lewis, Faber Paperback, 1981
A personal grief experience.

l) *Saying Goodbye to Your Baby*
by Priscilla Alderson, Still Birth and Neonatal Death Society (Sands)
Available from Sands at Argyle House, 29-31 Euston Road, London NW1 2SD

m) *Helping Children cope with Grief*
by Rosemary Wells, Sheldon Press

n) *When People Die*
by Williams & Ross MacDonald
'why do people die?' – 'what is death?'– 'facing loss' – 'helping others' – 'beliefs and rituals' – 'no easy answers' etc.

o) *The Great Blue Yonder*
by Alex Shearer, Macmillan, 2001
A helpful book about not having the opportunity to say 'goodbye'. The story explores the sudden death of a young boy.

17 PARENTS' SUPPORT GROUPS
Where to make contact with others

HeartLine has information on many useful organisations. Please contact our Administrator at the following address:

HeartLine Association,
Community Link, Surrey Heath House,
Knoll Road, Camberley, Surrey GU15 3HH
Tel: 01276 707636   Fax: 01276 707642
Email:heartline@easynet.co.uk
www.heartline.org.uk

OTHER CHILDREN'S HEART SUPPORT GROUPS IN THE UK:-
Here are some of the major organisations which may be able to help you. There are many local groups.
We recommend you to contact either HeartLine or CHF, whose address follows, to find your nearest support group.

CHILDREN'S HEART FEDERATION
Details of contact names and phone numbers are available from the office of The Children's Heart Federation,
52 Kennington Oval, London SE11 5SW.
Helpline Tel: 0808 808 5000
Tel: 020 7820 8517   Fax: 020 7735 8718
Email: chf@dircon.co.uk
www.childrens-heart-fed.org.uk

1. Contact a Family.
Brings together families of disabled children. Their parent adviser number

provides information about support groups and resources all over Britain.
209-211 City Road, London EC1V 1JN.
Tel: 020 7608 8700
Fax: 020 7608 8701

2. Action for Sick Children
3rd Floor, 300 Kingston Road, London SW20 8LX.
Tel: 020 7843 6444

3. ACT Association for Children
with Life Threatening or terminal Conditions and their families –
Orchard House, Orchard Lane,
Bristol BS1 5DT
Tel: 0117 922 1556   Fax: 0117 930 4707
Email: info@act.org.uk
www.@act.org.uk

4. ACE (Advisory Centre for Education)
offers information and advice on all aspects of state education.
1c Aberdeen Studios, 22 Highbury Grove,
London N5 2EA
Helpline: 0808 800 5793
www.ace-ed.org.uk

5. BLISS
Information and support for parents of premature or newborn babies (neonates).
Parents' Support Line (free): 0500 618140
Email: information@bliss.org.uk
www.bliss.org.uk

6. Child Poverty Action Group (CPAG) produces excellent publications on welfare rights and benefits (also available at libraries) and run an advice service for professionals, which is not open to the public.

The Child Poverty Action Group,
94 White Lion Street, London N1 9PF
Tel: 020 7837 7979   Fax: 020 7837 6414
Email: staff@cpag.org.uk
www.cpag.org.uk

7. IPSEA (Independent Panel for Special Education Advice)
A group of independent experts who give advice to parents who are uncertain or unhappy about the LEA's interpretation of their child's special needs.
6 Carlow Mews, Woodbridge IP12 1OH
Parent's Advice Line: 0800 0184016

8. TAMBA Twins and Multiple Birth Association.
Harnott House, 309 Chester Road,
Little Sutton, Ellesmere Port,
Cheshire CH66 1QQ
Tel: 0870 7703 304
Helpline: 01732 868000
Email: inquiries@tambahq.org.uk
www.tamba.org.uk

9. Down's Syndrome Association offers non medical help for parents of Down's Syndrome children, including leaflets and self help branches throughout the UK.
155 Mitcham Road, London SW17 9PQ.
Tel: 020 8682 4001   Fax: 020 8682 4012
www.downs-syndrome.org.uk

10. The Compassionate Friends provide support and help for people suffering the loss of a child by others who have been similarly bereaved. They have a telephone network and supply leaflets.
53 North Street, Bedminster,
Bristol BS3 1EN
Tel: 0117 953 9639
Helpline: 0117 953 9639
Email: info@tcf.org.uk
www.tcf.org.uk

11. Marfan Association
Rochester House, 5 Aldershot Rd.,
Fleet, Hants GU51 3NG
Answerphone: 01252 617320
Tel: 01252 810472   Fax: 01252 810473
Email: marfan@tinyonline.co.uk
www.marfan.org.uk

12. National Childbirth Trust
Alexandra House, Oldham Terrace, Acton
London W3 6NH.
Tel: 0870 4448 707

13. The Family Fund Trust
See Chapter 14 page 101 for more information.
PO Box 50, York, YO1 22X.
Tel: 01904 621115

14. Noonan's Syndrome Society
C/o Birth Defects Foundation, 'Martindale
Hawks Green, Cannock WS11 2XN
Tel: 08700 707020

15. The British Heart Foundation
14 Fitzhardinge Street,
London W1H 6DH
Tel: 020 7935 0185

16. GUCH Association
C/o 12 Rectory Road, Stanford-le-Hope,
Essex SS17 0DL.
A support group for adolescents and adults with congenital heart disorders.
Freephone Helpline: 0800 854 759
www.guch.demon.co.uk

18 MEDICAL TERMS
A Dictionary for Parents

Medical terms are often very confusing. Many of those that are frequently used in relation to children with heart problems are listed here with a brief explanation.

If there are any others related to your child that are used and you do not understand, please ask members of the team involved in your child's care to explain.

ABDOMEN – tummy

ABSCESS – a localised collection of infected liquid called pus.

ACCESSORY – Additional or extra

ACIDOSIS – loss of the normal balance of body chemistry resulting from poor heart action and poor blood supply to parts of the body.

ANAEMIA – reduction in the red blood cell count.

ANAESTHETIC – a chemical that produces loss of consciousness.

ANALGESIC – a chemical substance that produces freedom from pain.

ANEURYSM – a ballooning of the wall of a blood vessel or of the heart.

ANGIOPLASTY – stretching of a narrow artery by a balloon catheter.

ANOMALOUS – wrong

ANTICOAGULANT – a drug used to reduce blood clotting.

AORTA – main artery from the heart to the body.

AORTIC ARCH – topmost part of the aorta from which the head, neck and arm arteries arise.

AORTIC VALVE – the valve between the main pumping chamber and the aorta.

ARRHYTHMIA – irregular or abnormal heart action.

ARTERY – a blood vessel that carries blood away from the heart.

ASCITES – fluid in the abdomen.

ASYSTOLE – stoppage of heart action.

ATHEROMA – damage to the lining of arteries producing narrowing and reduction of blood flow onto which clots may form.

ATRESIA – blocked/missing/never formed.

ATRIUM – receiving chamber of heart.

AUTOPSY – examination of the body after death.

BANDING – an artificial narrowing of the lung artery with a 'band' or string to reduce blood flow.

BIFURCATION – division into two.

BIOPSY – removal of a small piece of tissue.

BLALOCK-TAUSSIG SHUNT – operation to join left or right subclavian artery to pulmonary artery.

BLOOD PRESSURE – the pressure of blood within the vessels.

BRADYCARDIA – slow heart rate.

BRONCHOMALACIA – softening of the cartilage supporting the bronchi.

BRONCHUS – main airway to each lung.

CAPILLARIES – very fine blood

vessels through whose walls food, oxygen, waste products, carbon dioxide are filtered to and from the body tissues.

CARBON DIOXIDE – waste gas produced as a by-product of body activity.

CARDIAC – heart.

CARDIAC OUTPUT – the amount of blood pumped by the heart per minute.

CARDIOMYOPATHY – disease of the heart muscle.

CARDIOPLEGIA – a chemical solution used to protect heart muscle during open heart surgery.

CARDIOPULMONARY BYPASS – a machine with a pump and an oxygenator to maintain blood supply to the body while the heart's action is stopped.

CATHETER – fine plastic tube to measure pressures or drain fluid.

CEREBRO-VASCULAR ACCIDENT – see stroke.

CHOLESTEROL – a fatty chemical found particularly in animal fat.

CHORDAE TENDONAE – fibrous cords that support the mitral and tricuspid valves.

CHOREA – spontaneous abnormal purposeless movements.

CHROMOSOMES – the basic protein that characterises each individual.

CHRONOTROPE – to increase heart rate

CLINICAL GOVERNANCE – A process in a hospital by which a committee of managers and doctors regularly review and maintain ethical standards.

CHYLE – a fluid containing a lot of fat within the lymphatic system.

CLUBBING – rounded swelling of the ends of the fingers or toes.

COARCTATION – narrowing in a blood vessel.

COIL – a device used for blocking blood vessels

COLLATERALS – natural additional blood vessels to help overcome a blockage.

CONDUIT – artificial tube.

CONGENITAL – present at birth

CONGESTION – too much fluid in a part of the body.

CONSOLIDATION – part of lungs becoming airless.

CONVULSION – a fit.

CORONARY ARTERIES – the blood supply to the heart muscle.

CORONER – an official who inquires into unnatural death e.g., sudden, unexpected or those related to procedures or operations.

CORRECTIVE – to return the circulation to normal.

CPAP – constant positive airway pressure, a way of keeping small airspaces open.

CYANOSIS – blue colouration of skin and lips owing to a lower amount of oxygen in the capillaries.

DEFIBRILLATOR – a machine to give an electrical shock used to treat abnormalities of heart rhythm.

DIALYSIS – a method of washing out waste products.

DIAPHRAGM – important muscle of breathing that separates the chest from the abdomen.

DIASTOLE – resting phase of heart action.

DIASTOLIC BLOOD PRESSURE – the lower of the blood pressure readings.

DOPPLER – the use of sound waves to assess speed and direction of blood flow.

DRAIN – a tube used to move fluid or air from the body.

DRIP – a means of getting food and drugs into a vein.

DUCT – a tube carrying fluid or blood.
DYSPHAGIA – difficulty with swallowing.
DYSPNOEA – breathlessness.

ECHOCARDIOGRAM – a picture of the heart and blood vessels using reflected high frequency sound waves.

ECMO – An abbreviation for "Extra Corporeal Membrane Oxygenation" a heart lung machine – which may be used to give medium term support for the patient's heart and lungs.

– ECTOMY – removal

ELECTROCARDIOGRAM – recording of the electrical activity of the heart.

ELECTRODES – fine wires that carry electrical activity from or into the heart.

EMBOLUS – an abnormal substance within the blood stream such as clot or air.

EMBRYO – the developing baby within the womb.

ENDOCARDIUM – smooth lining on the inside of the heart and its valves.

FAILURE – inability of the organ to cope with demands.

FALLOT'S TETRALOGY – combination of a hole between the ventricles, obstruction of blood flow to the lungs and a displacement of the aorta.

FAMILIAL – runs in families.

FEMORAL – related to the leg.

FIBRILLATION – disorganised heart contractions.

FLUTTER – abnormally fast regular beating usually of the atria.

FETUS – sometime spelt 'foetus' – developing baby within the womb.

FONTAN OPERATION – an operation to connect right atrium to lung artery

FORAMEN OVALE – small hole between the two receiving chambers.

GENE – an inherited characteristic, a part of a chromosome.

HAEMATOMA – a localised collection of blood outside a vessel.

HAEMOGLOBIN – the chemical carried in red cells that carries oxygen, carbon dioxide and gives colour to the blood..

HAEMOLYSIS – destruction of red cells.

HAEMOPTYSIS – blood coughed up from lungs.

HAEMORRHAGE – a leak of blood from blood vessels.

HEART BLOCK – a disturbance in the rhythm of the heart so that the ventricles beat more slowly then the atria.

HEART LUNG MACHINE – a machine that oxygenates and pumps blood around the body while heart operations are carried out.

HETEROGRAFT – (also called xenograft) – using a tissue from another species

HOMOGRAFT (also called allograft) – using tissue from another human.

HYPER – too much.

HYPERTENSION – elevated blood pressure.

HYPERTHERMIA – very high temperature

HYPO – too little.

HYPOTENSION – low blood pressure.

HYPOTHERMIA – very low temperature.

IDIOPATHIC – cause unknown.

IMMUNISATION – a method of increasing patient's defence against infection.

INCOMPETENCE – leaking.

INFANT – less than one year.

INFARCT – death of tissue related to blocking of the blood supply.

INFRA – below.

INFUSION – fluid or medication given slowly into a vein.

INOTROPE – a drug used to increase heart muscle function

INTRA – within.

INTUBATION – passage of a tube into the windpipe to assist with breathing.

ISCHAEMIA – reduction in organ function as a result of reduced blood supply.

-ITIS – infection.

JAUNDICE – yellow colouring of skin and eyes as a result of liver dysfunction or red cell breakdown.

JUXTA – nearby

KELOID – a hard lumpy scar from excess fibrous tissue.

LEUCOCYTE – white blood cell that fights infection.

LOBE – part of an organ.

LYMPH – body fluid running in channels, drains fluid and particularly fats from the bowel back into the circulation.

MACRO – large

MAPCAS – major aorto-pulmonary collateral vessels found in conditions like pulmonary atresia.

MEDIASTINUM – space in the chest between the lungs, heart and great vessels.

MICRO – small

MITRAL VALVE – two-cusped valve between the left atrium and left ventricle.

MONOCUSP – a single cusp from a donor valve.

MURMUR – noise produced by blood flow in the heart and vessels.

MUSTARD PROCEDURE – operation to redirect atrial blood flow.

NEONATE – baby in the first month of life.

NODE – area of specialised cell that controls the rhythm of the heart.

NUCLEUS – central part of most cells and contains the chromosomes.

OEDEMA – extra fluid accumulating in the tissue.

OESOPHAGUS – gullet

OLIGURIA – too little urine.

- OLOGY – the study of.

- OSTOMY – a hole.

- OTOMY – an incision.

OXIMETER – a machine to measure oxygen.

OXYGEN – part of the air that is needed by all animal cells for normal working.

OXYGENATOR – an artificial machine that delivers oxygen into the blood.

PACEMAKER – electrical control of the heart - natural/artificial.

PACING WIRES – wires that connect an artificial pacemaker to the heart.

PALLIATION – a procedure to improve the patient's condition.

PALPITATION – an uncomfortable sensation of heart beat which may be slow, fast, irregular or regular.

PARASYMPATHETIC NERVES – nerves to the heart that slow heart rate.

PARENTERAL – medicines or fluids given by injection.

PEDIATRIC – sometimes spelt 'paediatric' – word to describe science of medical problems in children.

PARESIS – paralysis.

PERI – nearby.

PERICARDIUM – lining bag in which the heart sits.

PERITONEUM – membrane lining the inside of the abdomen.

PHRENIC NERVE – nerve that supplies the diaphragm.

PHYSIOLOGICAL – functioning normally.

PLACENTA – part of the uterus that supplies the developing baby with nourishment and removes waste products..

PLASMA – liquid part of the blood.

PLATELETS – small particles in the blood which are important for blood clotting.

PLEURA – covering layer of the lungs and the inside of the chest.

PNEUMOTHORAX – air outside the lung and within the chest cavity.

POLYCYTHAEMIA – increased number of red blood cells.

PRECORDIUM – part of the chest in front of the heart.

PROCEDURE – another word for 'operation' or 'treatment'.

PROGNOSIS – an estimation of outlook for the patient's particular problem.

PROPHYLAXIS – prevention.

PROSTHETIC – artificial.

PULMONARY – the adjective used to describe lungs.

PULMONARY VALVE – the valve between the right ventricle and the lung artery.

PULSE – the arterial beat from forward blood flow produced by the heart contraction.

PUS – liquid produced by infection.

PYREXIA – high temperature.

RADIOGRAPH – photograph of part of the body using X-rays.

RADIO-ISOTOPE – a substance that gives off a small dose of radioactivity. It is used for diagnostic purposes.

RASTELLI PROCEDURE – operation to insert a conduit from right ventricle to lung artery.

RE-ENTRY-continual electrical reactivation of part of the heart

REGURGITANT – backward flow – leaking.

RENAL – pertaining to kidneys.

RESUSCITATION – a general term used to encompass treatment when the patient is very ill.

ROSS PROCEDURE – operation using patient's own pulmonary valve to replace an abnormal aortic valve.

SAC – bag.

SALINE – salt solution usually the same strength as body fluid.

SAPHENOUS – a vein in the leg.

SCLEROSIS – hardening of tissue.

SCOLIOSIS – curvature of the spine.

SEMILUNAR – crescent shaped, relates to the aortic or pulmonary valve leaflets.

SENNING PROCEDURE – operation to redirect atrial blood flow.

SEPTECTOMY – removal of a septum.

SEPTICAEMIA – an infection of the blood stream.

SEPTOSTOMY – a hole in the septum.

SEPTUM – a dividing structure.

SHOCK – severe failure of the circulation with cessation of normal body action.

SHUNT – a natural or artificial tube used to increase blood supply to the lungs.

SIGN – an abnormality found on examination.

SPHYGMOMANOMETER – instrument for measuring blood pressure.

STENOSIS – narrowing in the vessel or valve.

STENT– an expandable metal tube used to enlarge narrow vessels

STERNUM – breast bone.

STRIDOR – noisy breathing.

STROKE – loss of brain function related to blockage or bursting of its supplying blood vessel.

SUB – below.

SUBCLAVIAN – below the clavicle.

SUPRA – above.

SUTURE – fine string used to sew two parts together.

SYMPATHETIC NERVE – nerves to the heart that increase the heart rate.

SYMPTOM – complaint described by patient or family.

SYNCOPE – loss of consciousness related to lack of blood flow to the brain.

SYNDROME – a collection of abnormalities that together produce a recognisable pattern.

SYSTOLE – the period of contraction of the pumping chambers.

SYSTOLIC BLOOD PRESSURE – the top of blood pressure measurement taken when the heart is contracting.

TACHYCARDIA – rapid heart rate.

TACHYPNOEA – rapid breathing.

TAMPONADE – obstruction to filling of the heart by pressure from a surrounding collection of fluid.

THORACIC DUCT – vessel carrying lymph drainage from bowel through the chest to the subclavian vein.

THORACOTOMY – an operation on the chest.

THRESHOLD – lowest level of stimulus that will produce a response.

THRILL – vibration that can be felt, produced by abnormal blood flow.

THROMBOLYSIS – dissolving a clot in a blood vessel with drugs.

THROMBOSIS – clot formation.

THROMBUS – clot

TOXIC – an illness related to a poisonous by-product usually infection.

TRACHEA – windpipe.

TRACHEOMALACIA – softening of the cartilage that supports the windpipe.

TRACHEOSTOMY – a small tube inserted through a hole in the windpipe to assist ventilation.

TRANSPLANT – replace an organ by one from another person.

TRANSPOSITION – a change in the connection of chambers or blood vessels.

TRICUSPID VALVE – three leaflet valve between the right atrium and right ventricle.

TRUNCUS – single vessel arising from the heart that divides into aorta and lung artery.

UMBILICAL – tube that connects the placenta to the developing baby.

UNIFOCALISATION –bringing separate vessels together

UMBRELLA – a catheter device to block abnormal blood vessel

VACCINATION – used generally for immunisation.

VACCINE – a liquid of weak or killed micro-organisms, or their proteins that that can be used to prevent diseases.

VAD – Ventricular Assist Device to support cardiac function

VAGUS NERVE – nerve supply to the body and bowel, stimulation of which slows the heart rate.

VALVE – structure which allows blood flow in one direction and prevents leakage.

VALVOPLASTY – stretching of a narrow valve often with a balloon catheter.

VALVOTOMY – cutting or stretching of a narrow valve.

VASCULAR – relating to blood vessels.

VEGETATION – lumpy areas on heart valve caused by infection and blood clot.

VEIN (VENA) – thin walled vessel carrying blood towards the heart.

VENTRICLE – pumping chamber of the heart.

VASODILATOR – a drug to open up blood vessels

XENOGRAFT – tissue from another species

19 COMMON ABBREVIATIONS

From time to time abbreviations may be used both verbally and in written information. We list below some that may be of use to you.

ARP pathway	Anticipated recovery	N/G	Naso-gastric
ASD	Atrial septal defect	NHS	National Health Service
AVSD	Atrio-ventricular septal defect	NO	Nitric oxide
		NPU	Not passed urine
BNO	Bowels not opened	O_2	Oxygen
BO	Bowels opened	Obs.	Observations
BP	Blood pressure	OPD	Outpatient department
CHD	Congenital heart disease	PA	Pulmonary artery or pulmonary atresia
CICU	Cardiac intensive care unit		
CO_2	Carbon dioxide	PDA	Patent ductus arteriosus
CXR	Chest X-ray	PFO	Patent foramen ovale
DIRV	Double inlet right ventricle	PS	Pulmonary stenosis
DORV	Double outlet right ventricle	PU	Passed urine
ECG	Electro-cardiogram	RA	Right atrium
EEG	Electro-encephalogram	RV	Right ventricle
E/N	Enrolled nurse	S/N	Staff nurse
Hb	Haemoglobin	SVC	Superior vena cava
HLHS	Hypoplastic left heart syndrome	TAPVC	Total anomalous pulmonary venous connection
IVC	Inferior vena cava	TGA	Transposition of the great arteries
IVs	Intravenous infusions		
LA	Left atrium	TCPC	Total Caval Pulmonary Connection
Lines	Intravenous and intra-arterial cannulae	TOF	Tetralogy of Fallot or Tracheo-oesophageal fistula
LV	Left ventricle	VSD	Ventricular septal defect
NBM	Nil by mouth		

20 FILL-IN HEART DIAGRAMS

Your child's heart diagnosis

You may find it helpful for your consultant to use these pages to explain your child's heart condition.

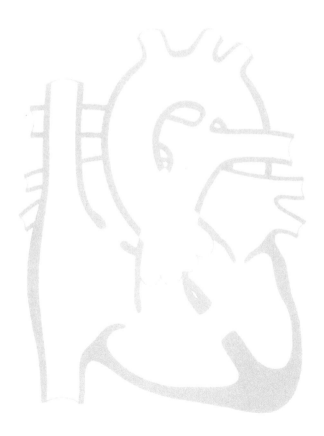

FILL-IN HEART DIAGRAMS

Your child's heart after correction

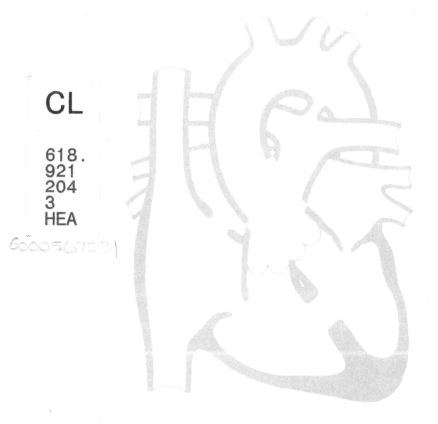